# New Earth Diet

Eat to Enlighten Yourself

# TONI TONEY

Copyright 2025
Toni Toney: All rights reserved.

This book may not be reproduced in whole or in part without written permission from Toni Toney except by a reviewer who may quote brief passages; nor may any part of this book be reproduced, republished, stored in a retrieval system, or transmitted in any form or by any means, electronic, mechanical, photocopying, recording, or other by any individual, organization or corporation without written permission from Toni Toney and New Earth Publishers.

DISCLAIMER: The nutritional and health information provided in this book is intended for educational purposes only. All efforts have been made to ensure the accuracy of the information contained in this book as of the date published. Nothing listed or mentioned in this book should be considered as medical advice or a substitute for medical advice for dealing with stress or any other medical problem. Consult your health-care professional for individual guidance on specific health issues and before following this or any program. Persons with serious medical conditions should seek professional care. The author and publisher specifically disclaim any liability, loss or risk, personal or otherwise, which is incurred as a consequence, directly or indirectly, of the use and application of the contents of this book.

Printed in the United States of America.
Book cover and layout design by keenankreative.com
Edited by Addison Fuller
First Edition
Published by: New Earth Publishers 2025

"In nature a curious yet simple phenomenon is often observed—a rise and fall. If perpetual, it alternates and becomes a fall and rise. Man has degenerated. This degeneration is due solely to his diet. He has fallen; but we hope that he has risen to the highest point in the art of shortening his days, and that in the present generation he will commence gradually to fall back on his original and ordained diet. Since the creation, the days of man's existence have been little by little decreasing—it has been a gradual fall; but both science and religion tells us that he must rise again, that his life on earth must be prolonged."

-Dr. Charles W. De Lacy Evans in "How to Prolong life," 1879.

## THE FALL
### *TO FORGET*

We are living in shifting times. The time to prepare our physical bodies for the shift of the ages is now—the shift from a fallen state of consciousness that tells you that you are just a physical body into an ascended state of consciousness that tells you that you are, in fact, PURE SPIRIT. The time has come to remember who and what we truly are!

## THE RETURN
### *TO REMEMBER*

The veil is lifting. We are waking up from a very deep sleep. The time has come to remember who and what we truly are. The only question is… Is your physical body ready to make this quantum shift in consciousness?

# CONTENTS

Endorsements .................................................. VI

What Is A New Earth Diet?................................ Vii

PART ONE ~ The Fall

~1~ The Illusion Of Separation...............................3

~2~ Our Body Our Earth ................................... 19

~3~ How To Create An Alkaline Body ................. 47

~4~ Nature's Food Chain ................................... 55

~5~ Eat Right For Your Anatomical Type............. 65

~6~ Dietary Devolution ...................................... 83

PART TWO ~ The Return

~7~ Enlighten Yourself With Nature's
Four "Fuel" Groups .................................... 119
Earth - Air - Fire - Water

Addendum................................................... 191

Reference Notes .......................................... 220

About The Author ....................................... 239

# ENDORSEMENTS

"This book is not just some new fad diet. It about our original diet as humans and what our diet should be now and in the future. It's about 'you are what you eat' and putting your personal health in the number one spot because without it, no matter what material wealth you have, you have nothing."

    –Smokey Robinson, Singer, Songwriter, Record Producer, and C-Founder of Motown

"Toni's knowledge on health and the body is invaluable. I am forever grateful for meeting her and learning the NEW EARTH ways for a healthier life in every way!"

    –Jenna Dewan, Actress

"After contemplating Toni Toney's internal acid rain theory, I performed a series of spinal taps on Alzheimer's, Parkinson's, and multiple sclerosis patients, as the cerebral spinal fluid is, in effect, the brain's water supply and should have a pH value of approximately 7.4. When I tested the cerebrospinal fluid's pH, to my amazement, she was right: it was approximately 5.5—the pH of environmental acid rain. Further dietary research is justified to see if shifting the pH of the brain terrain will provide clues in turning these devastating diseases around. From the evidence I now see I am optimistic."

    –Dr. Lorne Label, M.D., M.B.A, F.A.A.N. Associate Clinical Professor of Neurology, David Geffen School of Medicine, UCLA, Los Angeles

# WHAT IS THE NEW EARTH DIET?

When most of us hear the word "diet," we tend to think of a weight-loss program, which implies something we go on one day and off the next. Some may even think of it in the context of a health-care professional advising us to change to a healthier diet if our cholesterol or blood sugar is too high—just tossing out unhealthy foods and adding healthier choices to what we consume every day. So, when we hear in the news that we should add something like olive oil to our diet, it just means we should replace the trans-fat-laden hydrogenated gunk we're consuming with something healthier instead.

According to Merriam-Webster, however, the word "diet" means food and drink regularly consumed—a daily fare or habitual nourishment—a way of eating that people consume in specific countries or communities, such as the Mediterranean Diet, Japanese Diet, Italian Diet, and Turkish Diet. Then, we have the Standard American Diet—a habitual diet that most Americans consume that includes saturated fats, meat, dairy, and processed, prepackaged foods laced with excess empty calories, white sugar, white salt, white flour, and chemicals. We now know that this unnatural way of eating is why so many Americans are not only sick and tired but also suffering, more than any other country, from obesity, which is also why the weight-loss diet industry has exploded here.

The *New Earth Diet*, on the other hand, suggests a new way of eating that goes far beyond any of these narratives, especially the old "food science" narrative that focuses on the amount of fats, calories, carbohydrates, or proteins you eat every day. The New Earth way of eating is for those who instinctively know that a shift is occurring on planet Earth; that we are living in perilous times of biblical proportions.

It's a diet for those who are ready to raise the cellular frequency of their physical bodies, so they are prepared for the shift of the ages—the shift from a fallen state of consciousness into an ascended state of consciousness—the shift from the false perception that makes you believe you're separate from God, nature, and from everything and everyone around you. It's the shift from a physical state of consciousness back into the "Garden of Eden" spiritual state of consciousness where you once again remember who and what you truly are.

The only question that remains is...

*Are you ready to shift with me?*

# PART ONE
*The Fall*

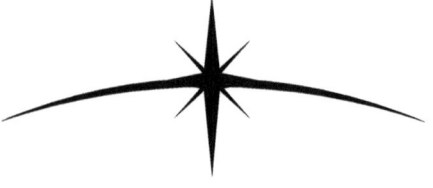

# — 1 —
# THE ILLUSION OF SEPARATION

A few decades ago, I became ill from a mysterious bacterial/viral infection that almost took my life. Unfortunately, the medical establishment had no cure for me. After being told that if my white blood cell count didn't go up in the next 24 hours, I started praying for a miracle. I had two young children who were much too young to lose their mother, so I began pleading with God for help. I had to live... if not for me, for my children!

As the stillness of the night wrapped itself around me, I closed my eyes and, for the first time ever, became consciously aware of the subtle breeze of my breath as it moved in and out of my nostrils.

Then suddenly, the same angelic presence that had appeared above me once before was once again hovering above me. We began having a felt-sense telepathic communication.

>I said, "I'm dying, and they have no cure for me!"

>The angelic presence replied, "How can they possibly have a cure when they don't understand your real problem?"

"So, what is my real problem?" I asked.

> The angelic presence replied, "The illusion that you're separate from God, from nature, and from everything and everyone around you. If you will but focus upon your breath, the breath of God who breathed you into physical existence, you will live!"

And so, I did. For hours!

The next morning, I woke up out of a deep, almost hypnotic sleep with a visceral knowing that it truly is the breath of God who is breathing me. God wasn't in a far-off place called Heaven judging my every move, as I had been taught. God was a subtle, yet dynamic power and presence within me!

A few moments later, the lab technician came into my room to take more blood. A few hours later, my primary care physician came in with the results. My family followed. He said…

> "I have no idea what happened in the night, but your white blood cell count is normal! It's a miracle!"

Screams of happiness filled the air of my once-isolation room.

Later that afternoon, as fate would have it, a close friend walked in, looked at my IV bag filled with antibiotics, hugged me, and said…

> "As Hippocrates said, you need to let food be your medicine and your medicine be your food!"

For the next few hours, he couldn't stop speaking about the father of medicine, Hippocrates (460 – c. 370 BC), and how he cured the sick with food.

He went on to say that Hippocrates based his entire healing practice on the observation and study of the human body; that a true physician was a teacher and the one who was sick was a student. To Hippocrates, the main duty of a physician was to teach their students the power of food to heal the body, then simply stand by and assist nature in performing its innate regenerative work. Hippocrates' goal was to empower his students by helping them understand that health is a natural effect of being in balance with nature and that disease is an unnatural result of being out of balance with nature.

To restore balance, Hippocrates trusted in nature to heal the body and the body to heal the mind. His prescribed medicines were whole plant foods, rest, enhanced elimination, fresh air, and sunlight. He also used intestinal purges and fasting to evacuate toxicity from the body, as well as the application of friction to increase circulation through rigorous massage and the use of hot and cold baths to further stimulate circulation.

He then began talking about Pasteur's germ theory versus Béchamp's Internal Terrain Theory to enlighten me about the germ that had threatened to take my life.

Antoine Béchamp, a nineteenth-century contemporary of Louis Pasteur, recognized that when the internal environment of the human body is in a healthy state of balance, germs do not have a breeding ground. Since germs feed off toxic waste, they simply cannot gain a foothold without a food supply. Pasteur and Béchamp each conducted prolific research into the cause of disease. Some say that they even worked side by side but came to very different conclusions.

Pasteur believed that the interior of the human body is sterile and static, like a spotlessly clean Petri dish. He believed that the cell is the elementary unit of life and hypothesized that harmful microbes were airborne and invaded the body from the outside in, causing such physical reactions as fermentation, putrefaction, and human disease. He taught that germs contaminate the tissue and cause disease; that we are the prey, and germs are the predators. This perspective is well known today as the germ theory.

Béchamp, on the other hand, believed that "disease is born of us and in us." He hypothesized that the cell couldn't be the elementary unit of life because certain microscopic entities within each cell had the ability to evolve into bacteria under certain conditions and change their form. This pleomorphic activity takes place depending upon the environment the cells live in. He named these microscopic entities microzymas. He found that microzymas, based on the environment the cells live in, could not only change their form, but their function as well, from helpful to harmful and back again, in countless variations.

While researching, he discovered that microzymas were so strong that he could not destroy them, even at the highest of temperatures. He even found live microzymas in limestone dating to a geologic period some 60 million years ago when the first mammals appeared on Earth.

What Béchamp discovered is that microzymas are present in the tissues and blood of all living organisms, where they remain benevolent and functional, especially as it pertains to cell division and immune function. He also discovered that when the welfare of the human body is threatened by the presence of potentially harmful material, such as an accumulation of undigested food particles and/or an accumulation of acids, a transmutation takes place.

The microzymas change their benevolent form into bacteria, viruses, yeast, or fungi, which immediately go to work to rid the body of this harmful material. Should the accumulated contamination continue to increase, the microorganisms would also continue to increase. But when the body's terrain's balance was restored, the bacteria, viruses, yeast, or fungi naturally reverted to the microzymas' normal benevolent state.

I was mesmerized!

After much research, Béchamp concluded that the real cause of disease was not the germ itself, but rather an internal terrain out of balance with nature and the natural order of things. Such imbalance is what makes the body a susceptible host to either external contamination or internal dissolution at the microscopic level.

Or, as Béchamp is reported to have said...

> "Living beings, filled with microzymas, carry within themselves the elements essential for health or for disease, for life or for death."

The choice is always ours!

Thus, his perspective was called the "Internal Terrain Theory," a theory that has never been refuted. It reflects the inner and outer message...

*That everything begins within us, and not the other way around.*

My friend believed that Béchamp's terrain theory was in complete alignment with how Hippocrates healed the body and, ultimately, the mind.

Even though my family thought I had become insanely delirious from the high fever, Béchamp's Internal Terrain Theory rang true to me, so I took my friend's advice and checked myself out of the hospital.

I was full of hope!

A few hours after I arrived home, my friend came by and delivered bags of organic produce. He had every fruit and vegetable imaginable. After decades of eating the Standard American Diet, it all seemed so strange to me. He also brought me a high-powered juicer and blender, along with an assortment of self-help books on the healing power of food and periodic juice fasting, as well as a book on how to cleanse accumulated toxic waste. I read all day and through the wee hours of the night.

Needless to say, my two children rebelled the next morning when I offered them a glass of carrot juice and a bowl of fresh fruit for breakfast instead of their usual glass of milk with a microwaved sticky bun. But I was on a mission, not just to heal myself, but to make sure my children stayed healthy as well.

For the next 90 days, I went on a sabbatical. Work took a backseat. I spent months creating recipes I knew my entire family would enjoy. I also read every book I could find on natural healing.

Not only did I take Béchamp's theory to heart, but I used Hippocrates' restorative method and healed my pain-ridden body with a diet of organic plant foods, fresh air, sunlight, juice fasting, and intestinal purgatives to evacuate the toxic wastes from my body. The totality of that experience caused insights to unfold within me that changed my life forever, preparing me for a destiny yet unknown.

Over the years, my desire for knowledge on how to achieve a perfect state of health took me all over the world. I traveled extensively, visiting and studying at various holistic healing centers where I received several certifications in the healing power of food and herbal detoxification.

My studies revealed that modern-day diseases increased as the contemporary American diet increased in net acid load relative to the diets of the ancestral pre-agricultural Homo sapiens. This shift most likely occurred because of the agricultural revolution and the ubiquity of processed grains and shelf-stable food products high in chemicals and devoid of essential nutrients. Then fad diets became the norm, the latest trend being a diet high in animal protein foods and low in phytochemical-rich plant foods that only come from fruits and vegetables.

Studies show that high-protein diets derived from meat and dairy increase net dietary acid load. Conversely, plant-based diets high in fruits and vegetables increase net dietary alkaline load. Over time, ingestion of a high dietary acid load can progress into a chronic low-grade level of metabolic acidosis.

The incidence of low-grade acidosis resulting from our modern diet has been well documented to cause health conditions such as osteoporosis, cancer, heart disease, kidney disease, and kidney stone formation. This chronic acid load creates a pH acid-alkaline imbalance, which in turn sets the conditions for "bugs" to show up on the scene, as their daily diet consists of waste! They are, in fact, nature's clean-up crew, and if you feed 'em, they're gonna' come!

After years of study and bringing my own internal environment back into a state of perfect pH acid-alkaline balance, I finally understood how the highly acidic foods I had been eating since my family moved off our farm and into town had created a toxic internal environment, which had become a perfect feeding ground for the pleomorphic germ that had threatened to take my life. As Béchamp had discovered, the germ was simply the effect of a toxic internal environment; it was not the cause.

> **Disease:**
> Dis ~ to move away from...
> Ease ~ the natural flow of life (freedom from pain and suffering)

So, if you've been tagged with the name of a disease, know that your real problem may just be a toxic, acidic internal terrain, caused by moving away from nature and the natural way of living!

## WE ARE ONE WITH NATURE

Nature, in its natural state, is lush, vibrant, and self-sustaining. Sadly, this is no longer true. Since the advent of the industrial age, over 100,000 unnatural chemical compounds have been created and spewed into the air we breathe, the fiery aura around the sun, the soil our food is grown in, and the water we drink. We have polluted our environment, our planet, and ourselves to a destructive end. We have literally and figuratively lost our way!

It is estimated that agricultural profits alone are now in the trillions of dollars every year from producing chemicals such as pesticides, with over one billion pounds of pesticides used in the United States alone every year, and approximately 5.6 billion pounds used worldwide.

This line of thinking is what brought the "chemical mafia" to my grandfather's farm so many years ago and sold him on the need to spray his lush green fields with chemical dust.

As a young child, I spent hours running barefoot and carefree in the green fields of my grandparents' farm, snacking on plump, heirloom tomatoes, strawberries straight off the vine, and raw carrots pulled straight from the dirt.

Back then, I was a very happy, healthy child, so full of life and the magical wonderment of nature. My grandfather grew acres of gardens, supplying our local community with lots of produce from his lush and thriving fields. Neighbors stopped by every couple of days, paid or bartered for what they needed, and exchanged stories of family and friends around my grandmother's long kitchen table.

The table was set every morning for family and farmhands to enjoy a big breakfast together before the workday began. Prayers were given in reverent gratitude for the food that was given so freely by the land for our nourishment. Communion around the table was the foundation from which our everyday living was woven.

Sometimes my great-grandmother and I would walk barefoot in the green fields for hours, communing with nature. I was told that Native American blood ran deep in her veins. Even so, she had a profound reverence and connection with Great Spirit and nature like no other. She was even able to see streams of brilliant colors radiating around the plants. At the time, I could see them, too.

Great-grandmother would often speak of Great Spirit as if it were her best friend. She explained that what most people don't understand is life force energy; that this dynamic energy is an extension of Great Spirit; that it exists within everything and everyone; and that this life force energy is what generates the streams of brilliant colors around plants and all that lives.

She would point out the various plant spirits around the plants and told me that plants have spirits, just like we do. She regarded plants as sentient, aware, intelligent, living healers, and would talk to them as though they could hear her.

She told me that I must always stay connected to Great Spirit and its life force energy; that Great Spirit's life force energy is what breathes my body, beats my heart, and knows how to heal me if I'm ever sick; that I must love and honor it with all my heart, mind, and soul. If I did, my life on Earth would be healthy and long.

But then one day, everything changed!

The notion of "better living through chemistry" had been planted in the soil of my grandfather's mind. The "chemical mafia" had convinced him of great profits if he would fertilize his fields and spray his plants with chemical dust.

Months later, I was warned that I could no longer run barefoot in the fields or eat my food from the vine or soil; that the chemical poisons could make me really sick.

As the mega-agribusiness profits rose and they gained more and more control over our land, my grandparents were forced to leave the family farm. Like the boiling frog myth, my grandfather had slowly been hypnotized into a very deep sleep. They soon joined the rest of the family in our small hometown. A few weeks later, my great-grandmother died. I believed it was from heartbreak.

Rather than pick our food from our lush green fields, we now bought chemical-laden food at the corner store. Instead of snacking on tomatoes or strawberries from the vine, or drinking water from a flowing stream, we were now eating candy from a wrapper and drinking soda from a fountain. The heirloom wheat I watched grow from seed to grain, milled from grain to flour, sifted and then baked into bread by the loving hands of my grandmother, was now pre-packaged white fluff, filled with preservatives and other additives.

Our eggs, once gathered from happy, healthy chickens that moved freely on the earth to their straw-filled nests, now came from drugged, semi-mutilated birds packed into overcrowded cages. The cattle that once roamed freely on our pastures were now herded into disease-ridden stockyards and fed food laced with artificial hormones and antibiotics. Animals were now forced to give their lives without the gratitude that was natural to my ancestors' way.

Sadly, we no longer communed around the table with friends and family, bartering goods or faithfully exchanging IOUs on a handshake and a hug. We had shifted from a tradition grounded in honor, community, and cooperation with nature, to one driven by control, productivity, and corporate profiteering concerns.

With today's rising temperatures and sea levels, facilitated in large part by the notion of "better living through chemistry," we could look back to the advent of industrialized agriculture, which coincided with the entire "industrial revolution" as the tip of the iceberg. Greed and the lust for power have led to the exploitation of resources without thought or concern for the welfare of those from whom these resources are taken.

But the destruction did not stop with our chemical-laden land and food; it continued in pharmaceutical laboratories. Grandmother's whole food plant extracts and herbal remedies had been replaced with pharmaceutical drugs, most often with side effects that were more noxious than the disease itself.

As time passed, our small neighborhood farm-to-market corner stores slowly disappeared into the shadows cast by large corporate conglomerates.

The late '50s saw the introduction of frozen TV dinners, ushering in a new era of "convenience," albeit with "inconvenient" yet-to-be-understood side effects. Frozen dinners quickly gave way to fast-food restaurants in the 60s, while the 80s saw the replacement of automobile service stations with 24-hour "convenience stores" stocked with everything anyone would need to eat on the run.

Through the seduction of television and the coercion of mass marketing, our children now believe that "real food" is cereal from a box, a hot dog on a bun, sugary glazed donuts, a burger with fries, a pizza with double cheese, deep-fried potato chips, or chicken nuggets washed down with a cola.

Because most of our children are now being fed a processed diet high in chemical-laden, non-nutritious junk foods, childhood obesity, along with its cascading related diseases, is at epidemic proportions. Most of our children's immune systems are failing them.

Every day, new microforms of virulent bacteria and viruses are spreading globally—an epidemic mostly fueled by the overuse of antibiotics. These microforms are highly pleomorphic, meaning they can change their form and evolve into even more aggressive ones.

Superbugs are also extremely intelligent and are already rendering our current medical methodologies for dealing with them ineffective. In the wake of the COVID-19 pandemic, an increasing number of authoritative voices are warning of the potential danger of a fungal species becoming the next plague to threaten humanity.

All of this should give us more than a pause—a pause that ignites a burning desire for a new way of living.

It seems that no matter where we turn today, we are confronted with yet another apocalyptic tide highlighting the error of our ways. Mounting news reports indicate that climate change is creating everything from droughts to record-breaking hurricanes, furious fires, mudslides, earthquakes, and tsunamis to acid rain and deforestation, and to the acidification of our lakes and oceans… all warning us that our plight is urgent.

We have poisoned our planet to the point where we are also experiencing unprecedented species extinction. Yet, as intelligent as we claim to be, we are also poisoning ourselves and our children to the point of extinction.

The pollution of our air, water, and soil is contributing to over 9 million deaths globally per year—approximately seven million of those deaths stem from indoor and outdoor air pollution. Sadly, our children are impacted by environmental pollution the most. It has been reported that approximately two million children are dying every year from environmental pollution.

In a study of newborns, researchers found 287 different pollutants in the blood of their umbilical cords: 180 of these toxins proved to be carcinogenic; 217 are known to be toxic to the brain and nervous system; and 208 cause birth defects.

All of this should give us more than a pause; that is, a pause that ignites a spark in our hearts and minds in favor of a new way of living—a type of resolve that promotes a change in the old ways of thinking in favor of new ones.

**The illusion of separation is our only problem!**

As time passed, I began to view nature through the eyes of oneness. We are not separate, as I had once believed.

I could now see that our planet's environmental crisis is but a mere reflection of our body's environmental crisis. How we are polluting our planet is the same way we are polluting ourselves. Like burning the wrong type of fuel (fossil fuel) in our planet's environment that adversely affects it, most of us are burning the wrong type of fuel (acidifying animal and processed foods loaded with toxic chemicals) in our body's environment that adversely affects it.

Albert Einstein said it best...

> "A human being is a part of the whole, called by us 'universe,' a part limited in time and space. He experiences himself, his thoughts, and feelings as something separate from the rest—a kind of optical delusion of his consciousness."

Thus, I have concluded that, in the end, most of our suffering—physically, mentally, emotionally, and spiritually—stems from the illusion of separation.

But the good news is...

*We are finally waking up!*

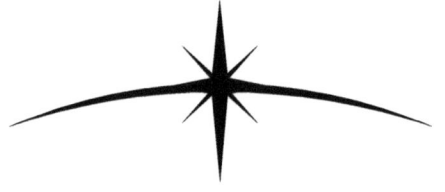

## — 2 —
# OUR BODY OUR EARTH

The belief that we are separate from nature has taken us down a very dismal path. It was during the time of Hippocrates that Greek philosophers observed the world around them and sought rational explanations for the origin and nature of the physical world and how interconnected everything is. Central to this worldview, they often divided the world into four elements: earth, air, fire, and water. It was through this model of the elemental world that Greek medicine took its stance...

> *The cause and cure of any type of physical illness are rooted in the larger conceptual viewpoint of the elemental world and our connection with it.*

This is because our physical bodies are also made up of mostly earth, air, fire, and water—the same classical elements of the world according to ancient Greek philosophy. Thus, how we thrive and how we die is, in part, the same.

The following chart shows the percentage of the primary elements in our bodies and the primary system that requires each element.

## OUR BODY'S ELEMENTAL COMPOSITION

| Element | % of Body Weight | Primary Systems Requiring This Element |
|---|---|---|
| Oxygen | 65 % | All Fluids, Bones, Teeth, Skin, Red Blood Cells, and Circulation |
| Carbon | 18 % | Teeth, Skin, Connective Tissue, Hair, and Nails |
| Hydrogen | 10 % | Blood and Cells |
| Nitrogen | 3 % | Muscles, Cartilage, Tissues, Ligaments, Tendons, and Flesh |
| Calcium | 2 % | Bones and Teeth |
| Phosphorus | 1 % | Blood and Brain |

Derived from H. A. Harper, V. W. Rodwell, P.A. Mayes, Review of Physiological Chemistry, 16th ed. (Los Altos, CA: Lange Medical Publications, 1977).
*Note: While there are numerous other essential minerals that comprise the human body, they are in concentrations of less than 1 percent, which is the reason they're not listed here.*

Interestingly, as you can see from the elemental chart, our physical bodies are made up of mostly oxygen. However, like the body of planet Earth, our bodies became one big body of water when oxygen and hydrogen merged in a particular way, making our physical bodies approximately 75 percent water! Interestingly, clean water is approximately 90 percent oxygen, and OXYGEN is the key to a healthy, sustainable life!

The question then becomes… what is the key to maintaining high levels of oxygen?

The key is—pH!

## The Power of pH

A new holistically minded medical perspective has emerged in our world today, which is...

> *Most every disease is intimately related to the pH of the fluids in our bodies.*

The fluid that is of most importance is called interstitial fluid, which is found in the spaces around the trillions of cells that make up our glands, organs, and tissues. It has been shown that virtually every degenerative disease such as diabetes, cancer, heart disease, joint pain, osteoporosis, arthritis, neurological diseases, skin conditions, and even tooth decay, has been directly associated with excess acids in our body's interstitial fluids, which are fluids that surround our cells.

> **An alkaline body high in oxygen is the key to a healthy, sustainable life!**

In practical terms, pH is a measure of the acidity or alkalinity of a water-based fluid. The pH scale runs from 0 to 14. A pH measurement of 7 is defined as neutral, being neither acid nor alkaline. Fluids with a pH measurement of less than 7 are acidic—the lower the number, the more acidic the fluid. Any number greater than 7 is alkaline—the higher the number, the greater the alkalinity.

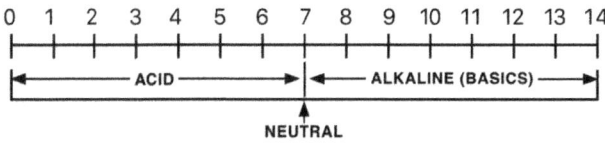

**The pH Scale**

The pH measurement of a fluid is directly related to the amount of oxygen it contains—the higher the pH reading, the more oxygen; the lower the pH reading, the less oxygen. Within the human body, our fluids should have a pH measurement of approximately 7.35-7.4, which equates to an oxygenated environment. If, however, the pH measurement of our fluids should drop below 7, a low-oxygenated environment ensues—the lower the drop, the lower the oxygen levels become.

Aerobic bacteria (or aerobes) are beneficial (good) bacteria that flourish in an oxygen-rich environment, whereas anaerobic bacteria are unbeneficial (bad) bacteria that flourish in a low-oxygen environment.

This is the KEY to understanding the power of pH and how we thrive and how we become sick and die!

In short, if our body's interstitial fluids—the fluids that our cells "swim" in—are slightly alkaline (7.35-7.4) and oxygen-rich, our cells and beneficial bacteria thrive, as do we! But if our body's interstitial fluids become acidic (6.5-5.5) and oxygen-starved, our cells and beneficial bacteria become sick and die, as do we!

> **Cell Death occurs in a toxic, low-oxygenated, acidic environment.**

Simply put, when enough of our cells and beneficial bacteria die, unbeneficial bacteria become the dominant force that sets the stage for almost every disease known. If this is allowed to happen, our bodies will painfully and slowly be reduced back into the dust of the earth!

**Unnatural Feeding: The Cause of Disease**
To better understand how bodies of water thrive and how they die, let's take a deep dive into how "unnatural feeding" disrupts the ecological balance of both our planet's and our body's waterways.

Let's begin by exploring the near-death of one of our nation's greatest bodies of water: Lake Erie.

Lake Erie, one of the most productive Great Lakes that divides Canada and the United States, was thriving and replete with aquatic life until surrounding industries and agricultural farms began "feeding" industrial waste, sewage, fertilizers, and pesticides into its waters. As a result, Lake Erie became saturated with high levels of unnatural nutrients such as phosphorus, nitrogen, and agricultural runoff. This type of "unnatural feeding" contributed to eutrophication—a process that encourages the development of algae blooms that create what's known as "dead zones."

Dead zones are areas within bodies of water where aquatic life cannot survive because of low oxygen levels caused by excessive nutrient pollution that reduces pH levels in bodies of water.

Unable to thrive in a low-oxygen acidic environment, dead fish began littering the shoreline, which led to massive fish kills. To compound an already ecological disaster, Lake Erie's waters became so polluted with oily petroleum-based sludge, and the gaseous products of rot and fermentation, that the surface of the lake literally caught fire!

This episode is what gave rise to the coining of a phrase which started to appear in national publications in the late 1960s...

"Lake Erie is dead!"

Fortunately, after the EPA stepped in and forced shoreline industrial and sewage plants to reduce the acidic nutrient dumping frenzy by eighty percent, the lake, over time, was restored.

This is why I say…

*Unnatural feeding is what causes most of our diseases!*

Lake Erie's fate is a perfect analogy for understanding how the human body thrives or how it becomes sick and dies. Like the trillions of fish and aquatic life that swim in the waters of our planet, we also have trillions of cells and beneficial microbes that "swim" throughout the waters of our body. At the microscopic level—our organs, glands, bones, skin, and tissues—every facet of our physical bodies is made up of cells. For our cells to thrive, ecological balance is absolutely everything!

> **To thrive, the water our cells "swim" in must be slightly alkaline and replete with oxygen.**

Unfortunately, most of us are continuously feeding unnatural acidifying foods loaded with toxic chemicals into the waters of our bodies. Interestingly, some of the most pervasive chemicals in the American diet are organic and inorganic phosphates, which are both extremely acidic.

Organic phosphates are mainly found in meat, eggs, dairy products, grains, and legumes. Inorganic phosphates are synthetic additives found in commercially produced sodas, baked goods, frozen dinners, processed meats, and junk foods of every kind.

Lastly, unnatural vegetable oils are added—all of which contribute to an ecological breakdown where our body's waters become an acidic, oxygen-deprived, inflammatory "lake of fire!"

When you begin to view the human body as a living, breathing ecosystem made up of earth, air, fire, and water, you, like me, will conclude that the "unnatural feeding" of acidifying foods into our body's waters is the same as the "unnatural feeding" of acidifying substances into our planet's waters—causing every ecological breakdown that we call disease!

This is why I deem myself an "internal environmentalist"… a person who studies the ecological life within the environment of both our bodies and our planet… a study that shows how we thrive and how we die!

**Candida and Algae**
Interestingly, Candida and algae are both unicellular and multicellular organisms. They live in small colonies throughout the waters of our planet and our bodies as an inherent part of our ecology. They are both polymorphic, having the ability to overgrow and change their form from beneficial to unbeneficial.

Everyone has Candida; it's part of the normal flora of the gastrointestinal and genitourinary tracts. Like algae, Candida is part of nature's food chain and will overgrow, or "bloom," to consume any excessive unnatural nutrients that are fed into the body. They are nature's cleanup crew—if you keep feeding them, they're going to keep blooming!

Eventually, if your unnatural feeding frenzy doesn't stop, the trillions of cells that "swim" in your body's waters will start to die due to an acidic, low-oxygen environment. As dead cells (like dead fish) start littering the shoreline of your tissues, a more aggressive, multicellular yeast/fungal form will appear on the scene, setting the stage for more serious conditions throughout different areas of your body.

Just as dead zones are created in the low-oxygen waters of our planet where aquatic life cannot thrive, dead zones can also be created in the low-oxygen waters of our bodies in much the same way. Such dead zones can be found in the areas of our body's organs, glands, and tissues.

This is why I say…

> *What we have long called disease is nothing more than a series of ecological breakdowns caused by unnatural feeding!*

These are the primary reasons that Candida can grow out of control:
- Unnatural feeding; that is, eating a diet high in acidic foods such as meat, dairy, and processed foods loaded with toxic chemicals.
- Eating a diet high in moderately acidic foods such as grains, beans, and processed foods.
- Drinking highly acidic drinks, such as sodas and sports drinks.
- An acidic, low-oxygen environment.
- Overeating.
- Taking drugs such as antibiotics and birth control pills, which

destroy the ecological balance of our beneficial microbial world.
- Stress, trauma, and emotional upsets.
- Your elimination organs (liver, kidneys, lungs, intestines, skin) being unable to efficiently eliminate toxic waste.

If left unchecked, the aggressive fungal form will grow into plant-like structures complete with roots that can break through the lining of your gastrointestinal wall, which can then break down the protective barrier between the intestinal wall and bloodstream. As a result, proteins and other food wastes that are not completely digested or eliminated can assault the immune system and cause tremendous fatigue, allergic reactions, and numerous other health conditions.

This abnormal, out-of-control growth allows Candida/fungus to travel to certain areas of your body, gaining a foothold in places where it was never meant to be. Thus, your ecological breakdown spirals!

While it generally goes undiagnosed, Candida/fungus overgrowth is an infectious silent killer—a destroyer of health, and the missing link in the understanding of modern-day diseases. But to believe that Candidiasis (a fungal infection caused by Candida) is the "cause of disease" is like saying "roaches cause a dirty kitchen!"

In short…

> *Candida/fungus is an inherent part of nature's food chain, and if you feed 'em, they're gonna' come!*

Candidiasis is known to cause many different symptoms and diseases depending on where in your body the overgrowth of Candida has colonized. If you are experiencing even a few of the following symptoms, you may have Candida overgrowth. If you have many of the symptoms, know that Candida has most likely been established in your body for a very long time.

**Candida-Related Symptoms and Diseases:**

- Allergies
- Autism
- Autoimmune Disorders
- Bad Breath
- Brain Fog
- Celiac Disease
- Chronic Sinusitis
- Chronic Fatigue
- Cancer
- Chronic Irritation
- Dermatitis
- Diabetes
- Depression
- Eczema
- Fibromyalgia
- Hair Loss
- Headaches
- IBS
- Intestinal Problems
- Itchy Red Eyes
- Jock Itch
- Joint Pain
- Low Immunity
- Low Sex Drive
- Low Adrenals
- Low Thyroid
- Migraine Headaches
- Oral Thrush
- Skin Fungus
- Skin Rashes
- Sinus, Ear, or Eye Infections
- Toenail Fungus
- Vaginal Yeast Infections
- Vision Problems
- Weight Gain
- Leaky Gut

If you have just one or two of the symptoms and you're not sure whether you have an overgrowth of Candida/fungus, the simple Candida Spit Test may help you confirm your suspicions, one way or the other.

This is an anecdotal home test that can be your first step to determine if Candida/fungus is well established in your body. It is called the Spit

Test basically because it is based on, well, your spit! To establish that it is yeast that is causing the saliva to test positive for Candida/fungus, it would be useful to eliminate all dairy for ten days before the test. It would also be useful to drink plenty of water for ten days before the test to make sure you are not dehydrated.

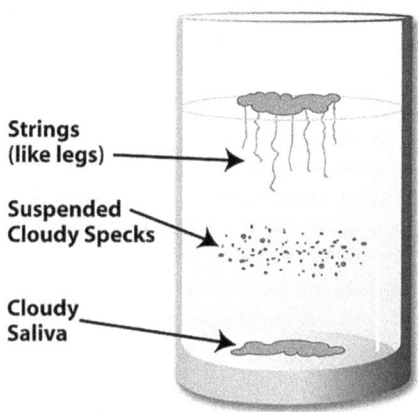

Once you have eliminated dairy for ten days and had adequate amounts of water for those same ten days, the steps for the Spit Test are as follows:

1. First thing in the morning, before you eat, brush your teeth, then swish your mouth with purified water.
2. Fill a clear glass with room temperature water.
3. Work up a dime-sized amount of saliva, then spit that saliva gently into the glass of water.
4. Leave the saliva for 30-45 minutes.

Now check it for one of the following:
- "String-like" formations coming down from the saliva at the top of the water.
- Cloudy saliva sitting at the bottom of the cup.

- Opaque specks of saliva in the middle of the cup.

Any of these three signs indicate that there is most likely a Candida overgrowth.

Because there's no real scientific research behind the Spit Test, to validate your suspicions, I also recommend a Karius blood test that can be ordered online or by your physician. This test can help you complete the invasive Candida/fungal infection (Candidiasis) puzzle.

An overgrowth of Candida/fungus is an S-O-S signal, warning you that your body is susceptible to various ecological breakdowns such as diabetes, cancer, and even neurological diseases.

### Diabetes: The Cause, The Cure

Let's consider what can happen if the waters of your body become overrun with Candida. Some so-called dietary authorities believe that eating a high-carbohydrate diet, or even natural sugar found in fruit, is what causes Candida to overgrow and may even be the cause of type-2 diabetes.

According to Dr. Doug Graham, author of *The 80/10/10 Diet*, Candida is a microbe that inherently lives in our intestines, tissues, and bloodstream. Candida's food is blood sugar, and when our blood sugar is present in normal amounts, Candida stays in balance and our internal environment thrives. The problem arises when our blood sugar becomes excessive, and Candida multiplies to consume the excessive sugar.

Unlike the traditional anti-Candida diet of no fruit and low carbohydrates, in his book, Dr. Graham concluded that a high fruit, high carbohydrate diet (the Genesis Diet we were originally designed to eat), with a very small amount of whole food fat from foods such as avocados, will not only stop the overgrowth of Candida, but over time, might even reverse it!

This dietary opinion is also echoed by Neal Barnard, M.D., author of Dr. Neal Barnard's Program for Reversing Diabetes, clinical researcher, and founding president of the Physicians Committee for Responsible Medicine (PCRM) in Washington, DC.

Dr. Barnard conducted clinical research with some 200 people who had type-2 diabetes, and what he discovered was monumental… they all had abnormal fat droplets inside of their muscle and liver cells, which had created insulin resistance.

Insulin resistance is the first stage of type-2 diabetes. Dr. Barnard found that when the membrane (skin) of our cells becomes clogged with fat, insulin—the hormone that escorts glucose into the cells—is unable to do its job, so glucose builds up in the bloodstream.

Some call this diabetes…

*I call it an ecological breakdown!*

Again, what inhibits insulin from escorting glucose into the cells for energy production is the unnatural accumulation of fat around our cells, which is ultimately caused by overeating unnatural fats and/or the liver's inability to break down fat efficiently. Even if you're eating whole food fats such as avocados, nuts, and seeds, over time, if your body isn't breaking them down properly, these undigested fats will also begin to accumulate around the membrane of your cells, blocking the transference of glucose.

The more fat you eat, the less effective insulin is at getting glucose into your cells and out of your bloodstream. Dr. Barnard's research proved that by eating a high-carbohydrate diet and eliminating every type of animal fat, you greatly reduce, and can even eliminate, the fat deposits in muscle and liver cells. While animal fat is the primary villain, vegetable oils, which are 100 percent unnatural extracted fat, are culprits as well.

In conclusion, Dr. Barnard's research found that a high-fiber, naturally low-fat, plant-based, vegan diet reduces insulin resistance, improves insulin sensitivity, reduces elevated glucose levels in the blood, and can even reverse type-2 diabetes!

## Cancer: The Cause, The Cure

Up until now, we have called one of our nation's most feared diseases—cancer—a mystery. But what if there's a tie-in between acidosis (too much acid in the body's tissues), low oxygen levels, Candida/fungal overgrowth, and cancer?

Let's explore

> "The cause of cancer is no longer a mystery—cancer is a fungus!"
> –Dr. Tullio Simoncini

In his book, *Cancer is a Fungus*, Italian oncologist Tullio Simoncini reveals that cancer does not develop out of some mysterious malfunctioning of the genes. This implies that cancer is intracellular (from within the cell), as most cancer researchers believe. Instead, Dr. Simoncini believes that cancer develops from a fungal infection and is, therefore, an extracellular (from outside of the cell) phenomenon. This is because fungus is always present in the tissues of cancer patients, especially in terminal patients.

From this standpoint, Dr. Simoncini is encouraging modern oncology researchers, who spend millions upon millions of dollars every year on studies that yield only minimally useful results, to move cancer research into the study of microorganisms such as fungus to solve the mysteries of cancer once and for all.

Sadly, at the time, the mainstream medical community rejected Simoncini's hypothesis, citing a lack of peer-reviewed studies that support it. Today, however, they have taken a second look! The American Association for Cancer Research has recently written that research does, in fact, show an association between fungi, including Candida, and cancer, but has not determined causation.

Once again, I call it…

*An ecological breakdown!*

As an "internal environmentalist," I believe that if medical research would look at the human body as a living ecosystem, made up of earth, air, fire, and water, they might conclude, as I have, that the underlying cause of an out-of-control proliferation of anaerobic fungus is an overly acidic, low-oxygen environment created by years of unnatural eating. As previously stated, Candida/yeast/fungus develops and overgrows in "dead zones" within acidic, low-oxygen areas of the body, such as our organs, glands, and tissues.

Therefore, as I see it...

> *It is an acidic, low-oxygen environment that creates an ecological breakdown we call cancer!*

As far back as 1924, Dr. Otto Warburg, who was a twice Nobel laureate, reported that the primary cause of cancer is the replacement of aerobic respiration (the inhalation and exhalation of oxygen) in normal body cells by anaerobic respiration (the conversion of food to energy without oxygen).

Dr. Warburg firmly believed that fermentation, the anaerobic conversion of sugar to carbon dioxide and alcohol by yeast, is the metabolic pathway of cancer cells. He discovered that this type of process is mostly associated with low oxygen levels, lactic acid production (a by-product of fermentation), and elevated carbon dioxide ($CO_2$) levels, as yeast cells give off $CO_2$ in their respiration, whereas normal cells give off oxygen in their respiration.

Dr. Warburg demonstrated that all forms of cancer are characterized by two basic conditions: acidosis (too much acid in the body's tissues) and low oxygen levels. He reported that acidosis and low oxygen levels are two sides of the same coin: where you have one, you have the other.

The link between acidosis, cellular oxygen deprivation, and disease was so firmly established in his mind that he altered his own way of life as a result. In his later years, Dr. Warburg was so convinced that disease was the result of acidosis and low oxygen levels that he would only eat organically grown alkaline fruits and vegetables, even though his colleagues deemed him a "health nut."

More recent research by Dr. Stephen Levine, molecular biologist and geneticist, and Paris Kidd, Ph.D., (Antioxidant Adaptation) indicates the likelihood that the switch from aerobic to anaerobic respiration in the cell is mediated by free radical damage. As the structure of the suffocating cell comes under attack from free radicals, and internal communication is impaired, the proliferating fungus takes over the function of energy production through fermentation.

Under normal conditions, a deeply damaged cell triggers its own death (called apoptosis)—a sacrifice to protect the larger community of the body. In saving the damaged cell, the fungus creates a monster—a monster we call cancer.

Here's what three other highly acclaimed medical experts have to say about the health hazards of an acidic, oxygen-deprived environment:

Noted German scientist and microbiologist Dr. Gunther Enderlein (1872–1968), stated...

> "Basically, there is not a multitude of diseases, but only one constitutional disease, namely the constant over-acidification of the blood... all of which is mainly the result of an inverted way of living and eating."

John McDougall, M.D., author of *The McDougall Plan: 12 Days to Dynamic Health*, reports...

> "Breast cancer is an environmental disease that has to do with the fats and synthetic chemicals in your diet."

Ed McCabe, M.D., and author of Flood Your Body with Oxygen: Therapy for Our Polluted World, says...

> "The bacteria, the viruses, the cancer cells, the fungus, the pathogens, almost all these microbes are anaerobic. Anaerobic is the scientific term that means they can't live in oxygen. So, I discovered over a hundred years' worth of research, actual medical history, going back documenting doctors that were using different oxygen therapies and products to reverse these low-oxygen conditions."

Mike Anderson, author of *The Rave Diet*, says...

> "The one thing an animal-based diet does best is kill people. It does this by clogging arteries and restricting the flow of blood and oxygen throughout the body. When you deprive the heart of oxygen, you get a heart attack. When you deprive the brain of oxygen, you get a stroke. When you deprive your tissues and cells of oxygen, you set up the underlying cause of all cancers."

From this standpoint, the cause and cure of almost every disease known may just hinge on the type of foods we are "feeding" into the waters of our body: acid or alkaline, processed or whole, easy to digest or hard to digest.

Always keep in mind that...

- Acidic foods, such as meat, dairy, and processed foods loaded with toxic chemicals, are not only hard to digest, but they also create an acidic, low-oxygen environment, which causes cell death and Candida/fungus to overgrow.

- Alkaline foods, such as fruits and vegetables, are not only easy to digest, but they also create an alkaline, oxygen-rich environment—a place where ecological balance is maintained, and our beneficial microbial world thrives.

Thus, the condition of your internal environment and the microbial world within you is what spawns life and health or death and disease. Microorganisms "gone bad" are simply a part of nature's food chain. They are reducer organisms, and the bottom line is…

*If you feed 'em, they're gonna' come!*

### Neurological Diseases: The Cause, The Cure

After researching the possible cause of neurological diseases such as Alzheimer's, Parkinson's, Multiple Sclerosis, and dementia, I discovered the results were one and the same: a systemic fungal infection caused by an acidic, low-oxygen environment. The area in which this ecological breakdown occurs is the brain.

Looking at these devastating neurological diseases through the eyes of an "internal environmentalist," here's how I came to this conclusion—a conclusion I call…

*The Internal Acid Rain Theory*

# THE INTERNAL ACID RAIN THEORY

Consider that acidosis has a pH value of approximately 5.5, as does acid rain. Acid rain is known to destroy everything it touches. Let's take a moment to consider the correlation between how acid rain destroys both our planet's and our body's ecosystems.

Acid rain forms in our planet's environment when unnatural acid-forming by-products are released into the atmosphere from certain industrial and agricultural practices, as well as from the burning of fossil fuels such as natural gas, coal, and oil. These acid-forming pollutants react in the atmosphere with water, oxygen, and other chemicals to form various compounds, resulting in an acidic residue or "ash" that is then carried through the atmosphere for hundreds of miles. As moisture condenses around the acidic ash, these compounds return to the earth by way of rain, snow, or fog. The effect is acid rain—an oxidative condensation that is defined as having a pH level of 5.5.

Acid rain forms in our body's environment when unnatural acid-forming by-products are released into our internal atmosphere when we "burn" the wrong types of food for fuel. These acid-forming pollutants react in our internal atmosphere with water, oxygen, and other chemicals, forming various compounds that result in an acidic residue or "ash" that is then carried throughout our body's internal atmosphere. As moisture condenses around the acidic ash, these compounds fall into the various ecosystems of our body. The effect is acid rain—an oxidative condensation that is defined as having a pH level of 5.5.

> Note: The formation of "acidic ash" is like burning wood in a stove, whereby oxygen unites with the wood to produce carbon

dioxide and water vapor that pass up through the chimney as smoke—the ashes remain in the stove.

As an internal environmentalist, I believe that when acid ash–forming foods are eaten, a type of acid rain is formed within us as bodily fluids condense around the acid ash that is left from the oxidative "burn." The acid ash can then travel throughout our body's internal environment, depositing its destructive ash throughout the various ecosystems of our body—just like acid rain deposits its destructive ash throughout the various ecosystems of our earth.

What I am proposing is that a type of internal acid rain, caused by burning the wrong type of foods for fuel in our body's internal environment, is the beginning stage of almost every neurological disease known.

Let's now consider three similarities between how acid rain destroys our earth's trees and how it also destroys our body's tree:

## (1) Our Earth's Trees
A tree has branches that are insulated with a waxy protective coating, which protects the tree from any type of environmental threat, i.e., weather or opportunistic "bugs." But if acid rain falls on its branches, its acidic burn will break down its protective coating, thus exposing the tree to environmental threats and weakening the tree's immunity.

## Our Body's Tree
Similarly, the human body has a tree called the spinal column. Our spinal column also has branches called nerves that are covered with a waxy protective coating known as the myelin sheath. This fatty

protective coating also shields our branches (nerves) from any type of environmental threat. In the same manner that acid rain breaks down the waxy protective coating on the branches of the earth's trees, internal acids can also break down the myelin sheath from around our nerves.

### (2) Our Earth's Trees

A tree has a root system with tiny hairs that reach out into the soil of the earth. These hairs are responsible for extracting, absorbing, and transferring nutrients into the tree. Mostly unseen by the human eye, there are billions of microorganisms that inhabit the upper layers of the soil. Within nature's food chain, these microorganisms are responsible for breaking down dead organic matter into compounds that provide the nutrients necessary for plant growth. But when acid rain falls onto the earth, it not only destroys the host of living microorganisms within the upper layers of the soil, but it also depletes the nutrients from the soil, causing a decline in plant growth and further weakening the immunity of the tree.

### Our Body's Tree

Similarly, just as a tree has roots with fine hairs that reach out into the soil for nutrients, we have an inverted root system called the intestinal tract equipped with tiny hairs called villi. These hairs are responsible for extracting, absorbing, and transferring nutrients into various areas of our bodies. Like a tree has billions of beneficial microorganisms that live in the soil, we also have billions of beneficial microorganisms that live in our intestinal tract. The job of these microorganisms is to break down the foods we eat into absorbable nutrients. Sadly, these microorganisms are destroyed by the onslaught of acid ash-forming foods.

## (3) Our Earth's Trees

The soil that a tree is rooted in contains heavy metals such as aluminum, mercury, and cadmium, which are normally bound in the soil, but are unbound and released into the soil by the onslaught of acid rain. These toxic metals are then absorbed through the tiny hairs of the tree's root system, making it difficult for trees to take up water and nutrients necessary for the tree's health. Over time, the tree's root system weakens and breaks down, causing decaying matter to build up inside the root. The tree completely loses its immunity as it begins to rot and decay. This is when an army of reducer organisms will show up on the scene to reduce what's dead and dying back into the dust of the earth!

So instead of using "pesticides" to kill the bugs we call the enemy, perhaps we should ask…

*Why have these bugs arrived on the scene?*

## Our Body's Tree

Similarly, our intestinal tract is further destroyed when heavy metals such as aluminum, mercury, and cadmium are released into its environment. These toxic metals are taken up by the villi, which inhibits the mucous lining of our intestines from absorbing water and nutrients necessary for our body's overall health. Over time, as our intestinal tract weakens and breaks down, unabsorbed water and undigested food particles build up, which can ultimately cause "leaky gut syndrome." If our gut leaks, toxins can be released into our bloodstream, which may be responsible for a huge variety of health issues, ranging from minor (bloating, cramps, fatigue, food allergies and sensitivities, gas, and headaches) to bigger health issues such as autoimmune conditions, depression, diabetes, and inflammatory bowel diseases. If our intestinal tract's immunity continues to weaken, reducer organisms such as bacteria, yeast, fungus, and mold will arrive on the scene to decompose what is dead and dying back into the dust of the earth.

So instead of using "antibiotics" to kill these bugs we call the enemy, perhaps we should ask…

*Why have these bugs arrived on the scene?*

**Validation of My Internal Acid Rain Theory**
To validate my internal acid rain theory, neurologist Lorne Label, M.D., conducted pH studies on some of his patients who had been stricken with neurological diseases. We had discussed the latest medical research that revealed Chlamydia bacteria could be the cause of these devastating diseases, as they were almost always present in those suffering from Parkinson's, Alzheimer's, and multiple sclerosis.

Agreeing with me that bacteria were opportunistic and are most likely not the originating cause of these devastating diseases, he decided to perform several spinal taps on some of his neurologically concerned patients to test the pH of their cerebrospinal fluid.

About a month later, Dr. Label reported back…

> "After contemplating Toni Toney's internal acid rain theory, I performed several spinal taps on Alzheimer's, Parkinson's, and multiple sclerosis patients, as the cerebrospinal fluid is, in effect, the brain's 'water' supply and should have a pH value of approximately 7.4. When I tested the cerebrospinal fluid's pH, to my amazement, she was right: it was approximately 5.5—the

pH of environmental acid rain. Further research is justified to see if shifting the pH of the brain terrain will provide clues in turning these devastating diseases around. From the evidence I now see, I am optimistic."

Interestingly, there's an increasing number of authoritative voices warning of the potential danger of a fungal species becoming the next plague to threaten humanity.

According to The National Library of Medicine (NIH), fungal infections of the central nervous system (CNS) have become significantly more common over the past two decades. Invasion of the CNS largely depends on the immune status of the host and the virulence of the fungal strain. Infections with fungi cause significant morbidity in immunocompromised hosts, and the involvement of the CNS may lead to fatal consequences.

Could it be that…

> *The cause* is a toxic, overly acidic, low-oxygen internal environment mostly caused by unnatural eating—foods such as meat, dairy, and processed foods loaded with toxic chemicals—a diet that destroys the beneficial microbial world within us and prevents us from experiencing our natural healthy state of being!

> *The cure* is a clean, alkaline, oxygen-rich internal environment mostly caused by natural eating—plant foods such as fruits and vegetables—a diet that supports the beneficial microbial world within us and keeps us connected to our natural healthy state of being!

Therefore, to turn any internal environmental crisis that you may be facing around, keep in mind that unnatural eating is what spawns our body's bacterial world to produce life and health or disease and death. The ecological balance of your internal environment is, therefore, the key to living a healthy, vibrant life!

Always remember that...

> *An alkaline environment replete with oxygen creates an environment where health thrives, and disease dies!*

This is why I have long said...

> *Alkalizing is absolutely everything!*

## THE FOUR STAGES OF ACIDOSIS

As I see it, ecological breakdowns caused by unnatural eating and living are at the root cause of most every degenerative disease and progress through four distinct ecological breakdown stages.

### STAGE 1: Autointoxication

Autointoxication takes place when we constantly burn unnatural acid foods and other acidifying substances into our body's internal environment. Over time, as acid ash and toxic waste accumulate, our internal environment becomes overly acidic, our microbial world is disturbed, our oxygen levels lower, and our organs and glands become congested, sluggish, and ineffective at performing their jobs.

Some of the physical and emotional conditions associated with this first stage of internal acidity are low energy, mild depression, muscle tension, digestive disorders, headache, sore throat, irritability, skin eruptions, kidney or bladder infection, muscle aches, bloating, anxiety, hypoglycemia, short attention span, hyperactivity, confusion, sinus pressure, mucous drainage, weight gain or loss, nightmares, hypersensitivity, or emotional volatility. Over time, if acids and toxic wastes are not properly eliminated, they settle deeper into the tissues, causing more serious conditions to develop depending on the area in which they reside.

## STAGE 2: Autoimmunization

Autoimmunization takes place when the immune system begins a self-attacking, misdirected response to the continual accumulation of toxic chemicals, undigested waste, and acid ash throughout the blood, lymph, and tissues of our body. The immune system becomes so compromised that it is unable to prevent the assault of pathogenic microorganisms. If this assault is not dealt with, an inflammatory response is triggered by the immune system in an attempt to repair the damage.

Chronic symptoms progress toward environmental or food allergies, migraine headaches, high blood pressure, irritable bowel syndrome, leaky gut, acid reflux, celiac disease, Crohn's disease, high cholesterol, asthma, sinus infections, lupus, chronic fatigue syndrome, fibromyalgia, kidney stones, gallstones, Parkinson's, Alzheimer's, multiple sclerosis, bronchial pneumonia, arthritis, depression, obesity, addictions, and diabetes.

**STAGE 3: Autoinfection**
Autoinfection takes place with the proliferation of pathogenic microorganisms in a highly acidic, toxic, low-oxygen environment. Cell death accelerates, and the body is now in a full-blown state of chronic acidosis. Systemic Candida and fungal infections rage out of control. The body's immunity becomes overwhelmed in its attempt to sustain ecological balance. If this ecological breakdown is not dealt with, the automatic immune response is unremitting reinfection with larvae produced by parasites and worms. In essence, the undertakers have arrived on the scene.

Some of the physical conditions associated with this advanced stage of acidification are heart attack, cancer, AIDS, and advanced expressions of stage-two autoimmune conditions.

**STAGE 4: Auto-Predictable Death!**
So instead of calling your disease a medically assigned name, why not consider the fact that you may just be experiencing an ecological breakdown caused by unnatural eating? Maybe then you can finally let go of the theory that germs are your enemy and take hold of the truth behind what the philosopher Pogo once said…

"We have met the real enemy, and the enemy is us!"

# — 3 —
# HOW TO CREATE AN ALKALINE BODY

As previously stated, our physical bodies are made up of trillions of cells that swim throughout your body's "watery terrain." The importance of the condition of our internal environment in which our cells exist in cannot be understated. Water plays a crucial role in maintaining the balance of nutrients, waste removal, and communication between cells. In a way, the condition of the "water" in our bodies determine how well those cells function and whether they thrive, deteriorate, or die!

This knowledge is a perfect reminder of how interconnected everything is, and how essential basic things like proper hydration, pH balance, and overall fluid homeostasis are to our health and overall wellbeing.

**Blood and Lymph—The Lifeblood of Cellular Health**
Our bodies are made up of two fluids—blood and lymph—with trillions of cells. While most of us have been taught that we have "blood" that flows throughout a very complex circulatory system (arteries and veins), what most of us haven't been taught is that we have another fluid called "lymph" that flows throughout another complex system

(lymphatic vessels) known as the lymphatic system. The startling fact is that we have twice as much lymph fluid than blood!

While blood "nourishes" our body's trillions of cells, lymph "carries" away cellular metabolic wastes. Cellular wastes, which are acidic, are then eliminated from the body via the kidneys, colon, skin, and other associated eliminatory processes. In essence, our cells eat and cells poop!

But what happens if our cells aren't properly "nourished" and if acidic cellular waste isn't "eliminated" properly? Over time, our entire body becomes one big malnourished, toxic mess. This malnourished, toxic mess is what medical science calls… "disease!"

> Dis – To move away from
> Ease – The natural flow of life
> (freedom from pain and suffering)

According to Robert Morse, N.D., D.Sc., M.H., lymphatic congestion (acid stagnation) and acidosis (the accumulation of acidic wastes) is the underlying cause of our body's degenerative health issues. He believes that lymphatic congestion is the underlying cause for most every disease known.

Lymphatic congestion begins when the kidneys (which are like a sponge) are overloaded with waste and are unable to eliminate waste properly. Poor kidney function is the result of eating a long-term acidic diet of meat, dairy, and processed foods… all low in *ELECTROLYTES*.

## Electrolytes—Tiny but Mighty

The importance of electrolytes in maintaining cellular health is a game-changer for understanding our health. Electrolytes are specific minerals that break down into tiny, electrically charged particles called ions. Ions are molecules that hold an electrical charge, when they dissolve in water. These ions carry electrical energy necessary for many bodily functions.

Every fluid and cell in your body contains electrolytes. They help your body regulate chemical reactions, maintain the balance between fluids inside and outside your cells, maintain blood pH levels, and so much more. Young or old, athletic or sedentary, electrolytes play a crucial role in some of the body's most vital functions.

But what exactly are these mysterious substances, and why are they so vital to our cellular health? Let's explore why these tiny but mighty electrolytes are so essential:

- Nerve Function: They transmit electrical signals between nerve cells, enabling critical tasks like reflexes and sensory perception.
- Muscle Contraction: Ever had a muscle cramp? That's often due to an imbalance of electrolytes. Proper balance helps muscles contract and relax smoothly.
- Hydration: Electrolytes help regulate the balance of fluids in and out of cells, tissues, and organs, keeping you hydrated.
- Heart Function: Your heart's rhythmic beating is orchestrated by these small particles. An imbalance can lead to severe heart issues.
- Acid-Alkaline Balance: Electrolytes help maintain the optimal pH level in your body, ensuring that it's neither too acid nor

alkaline. pH is a scale that measures whether a fluid is an acid or alkaline.

As previously stated, our body's natural blood pH is between 7.36 and 7.44 as is your lymph. Acids have a pH level of less than 7. Neutral has a pH level of 7. Alkaline has a pH of more than 7.

The significance of electrolytes to maintain proper pH balance cannot be overstated. From the rhythm of our heartbeat to the simple pleasure of a refreshing drink, these microscopic electrolytes are working tirelessly to keep us healthy and hydrated.

So whether through consuming electrolyte-rich foods, such as raw fruits and veggies or adding coconut water to your routine, embracing the power of electrolytes cannot be overstated. They are the primary key to you experiencing optimal health.

You may be wondering… so what's the difference between minerals and electrolytes? The basic difference is that minerals are a broad category of elements that can be electrically charged or uncharged, while electrolytes are minerals that have an electrical charge when dissolved in water.

In essence, electrolytes are minerals, but not all minerals are electrolytes. Minerals are a category of micronutrients that naturally occur in our environment and have unique health benefits. There are 16 dietary minerals, six of which are also electrolytes: sodium, potassium, calcium, magnesium, chloride, and phosphorus.

## The Four Main Electrolytes

As previously stated, electrolytes are integral to our body's function, but do you know what the four main champions are that regulate your chemistry? Let's narrow our focus and dive into the four electrolytes that make all the magic happen:

- ✓ Sodium and Potassium
- ✓ Calcium and Magnesium

From the balance of fluids to the rhythm of your heart, to maintaining proper blood pH levels, these four vital electrolytes work tirelessly behind the scenes to keep you at your best.

Here's a closer look at these four essential electrolytes:

**Sodium:** Sodium from plant foods is extremely important in the body because it plays a crucial role in fluid regulation, maintaining proper blood pressure, supporting nutrient transport, and contributing to muscle and nerve function; ensuring adequate sodium intake from plant sources helps to maintain overall bodily balance and prevent complications associated with sodium deficiency, medically known as hyponatremia.

**Plant foods that are the highest in sodium are:**
Celery, beet, spinach, artichoke, broccoli, carrot, radish, sweet potato, kale, Brussel sprouts, spaghetti squash, turnip, collard greens, cauliflower, asparagus, lettuce, parsnip, potato, cabbage.

**Potassium:** Potassium from plant foods is crucial for the body because it acts as an electrolyte, helping to regulate fluid balance, support proper nerve and muscle function, maintain a healthy heartbeat, and can contribute to lowering blood pressure, especially when paired with a diet low in sodium; making it vital for overall health and particularly important for managing cardiovascular health.

**Plant foods that are the highest in potassium are:**
Bananas, avocadoes, dried fruits (raisins, apricots), spinach, broccoli, beet greens, pomegranates, cantaloupe, oranges, tomatoes, beans, lentils, potatoes, acorn and butternut squash.

Together, sodium and potassium play a crucial role in maintaining proper fluid balance within the body. Sodium is primarily responsible for extracellular fluid (outside the cell) and potassium is primarily responsible for intracellular fluid (inside the cell).

Essentially, sodium and potassium work in tandem through what's called, "the sodium-potassium pump" (a protein embedded in cell membranes that actively moves sodium ions out of the cell and potassium ions into the cell) to ensure proper cell function by regulating your acid/alkaline balance and overall bodily processes.

**Calcium:** Your body needs calcium for muscles to move and for nerves to carry messages between your brain and every part of your body. Calcium also helps blood vessels move blood throughout your body and helps release hormones that affect many functions in your body. It is also needed to build strong bones! Vitamin D helps your body absorb calcium.

**Plant foods that are the highest in calcium are:**
Dark green leafy vegetables, broccoli, kale, Bok choy, beans, lentils, figs, oranges, seaweed, black strap molasses, nuts and seeds such as almonds, Brazil, poppy, pumpkin, sesame, celery, and chia, culinary

dried or fresh herbs such as basil, marjoram, and sage.

**Magnesium:** Your body needs magnesium for many processes, including regulating muscle and nerve function, blood sugar levels, blood pressure and aiding in overall energy production.

**Plant foods that are the highest in magnesium are:**
Spinach, Swiss chard, collard greens, quinoa, black beans, lima beans, green peas, sweet corn, potatoes, flaxseeds, pumpkin and chia seeds, avocadoes, almonds, cashews, papaya, bananas, blackberries, and best of all… dark chocolate (70%-85% cocoa).

From your bones to your blood, the dynamic duo between calcium and magnesium works synergistically to support various physiological functions, including bone health, muscle function, nerve transmission, and cardiovascular health. Calcium makes muscles contract, while magnesium is good for relaxation, which is why magnesium is good for sleep. Together, these two minerals regulate the heartbeat. Electrical impulses provoke the calcium within the cells of the heart muscle, stimulating a contracting movement.

It is important to understand that these four main electrolytes are the backbone of critical functions, such as regulating proper pH balance, throughout your entire body. Therefore, ensuring that you get enough of them is the key to living a long, healthy, vibrant life!

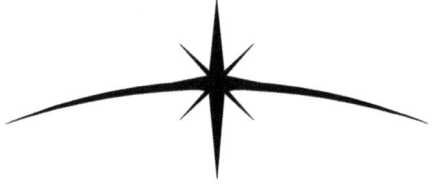

# — 4 —
# NATURE'S FOOD CHAIN

To understand nature's food chain is to know how to live a sustainable life on Earth. Within the realm of ecology, the food chain illustrates how energy and nutrients are transferred from one living organism to another in the form of food. As you'll soon learn, the food chain is an elegant, systematic arrangement that builds upon itself so that it can supply all living things with the amount of energy they need based on their size, activity, and lifestyle.

In the end, the food chain becomes a cycle of life in which all energy sources break down to feed the earth, then the cycle begins once again, and life continues. This cycle is how nature beautifully orchestrates the natural rhythms of self-sustaining ecosystems.

Within the hierarchy of the food chain, each group of species feeds on the group below it, each benefiting from the chemical energy of photosynthesis. As an example, humans benefit from the sun's energy by eating fruits from trees and plants from the earth that are produced through photosynthesis. Animals are the same, in that they either consume plants as a primary source of fuel or they consume other animals that consume plants. Basically, no matter where a species fits within the food chain, if they are "naturally feeding," they are consuming, at varying degrees, food that has the sun's energy.

This way of natural feeding can be used to divide every living creature within an ecosystem, including humans, into one of three categories: (1) producer organisms, (2) consumer organisms, and (3) reducer organisms.

- Producer organisms produce food for other species.
- Consumer organisms consume food.
- Reducer organisms (also known as decomposer organisms) convert previously living creatures back into organic matter.

To follow the wisdom of natural feeding held within the hierarchy of nature's food chain is the key to living a prosperous, healthy, long life on earth.

## PRODUCER ORGANISMS

Producers are organisms that make their own food. Within planetary food chains, they are plants, trees, bushes, grasses, and anything that has leaves. They are called autotrophs (from Greek, "auto" means "self" and "troph" means "feeding") because they create energy by absorbing carbon dioxide from the air through their leaves and sucking up water and nutrients from the soil with the help of fungi and bacteria. They use the sun's energy to convert carbon dioxide into oxygen and water vapor, which they then release through their leaves into the atmosphere. They create energy in the form of glucose (a type of sugar), amino acids, proteins, and fats, which they store inside new cells that are made using the nutrients (nitrogen, sulfur, and phosphate) they took from the soil. Thus, they are responsible for infusing energy into the food chain, making them the first link of the food chain. Without green plants, all the other animals in the food chain would not exist.

# CONSUMER ORGANISMS

Consumers cannot make their own food. They must consume other living things to obtain energy. Consumers are also called heterotrophs (from Greek, "hetero" means "other" and "troph" means "feeding"). There are different types of consumers defined by the type of food that they need to consume to produce energy:

**Primary Consumers**
Primary consumers eat producers. They are the next link in the food chain. There are two categories:

> (1) Herbivores: Primary consumers are usually herbivores—animals that feed on plants. They can be as small as grasshoppers and hummingbirds or as large as deer and cows. They typically have multiple stomach chambers and complex digestive systems, including long intestinal tracts, which are designed to maximize the energy they can absorb from the plants they consume. Herbivores are important energy sources for secondary consumers who benefit from the energy they produce and store inside their bodies.

> (2) Frugivores: Humans and primates are also called primary consumer organisms because they acquire their energy primarily from consuming fruit, along with some nuts, seeds, and green leaves, instead of grasses. (For more detailed information, please refer to Chapter 4).

**Secondary Consumer Organisms**

Secondary consumers eat primary consumers, making them the next link in the food chain. There are two categories:

> (1) Carnivores: Carnivores are animals such as owls, vultures, wolves, and bobcats. They are called secondary consumer organisms because they derive their energy from eating the flesh of herbivores. Their digestive systems do not efficiently or effectively process a plant-based diet. They have less complex digestive systems and shorter intestinal tracts than herbivores.
>
> (2) Omnivores: Omnivores are animals such as opossums, pigs, bears, chickens, emus, and a variety of birds. They eat plant foods, seeds, and meat for their nourishment, which is why they're often called mixed consumer organisms. This category would also include fish, as some fish consume algae and various other plants while others are more carnivorous. Their digestive systems can process both plants and animals. This feeding strategy is a great advantage when food is scarce because omnivores benefit from the greatest variety of food sources.

## REDUCER ORGANISMS

Microorganisms such as bacteria, Candida/yeast/fungi, parasites, and algae are the end of the food chain. They are called reducer organisms, or decomposers, because their inherent function is to scavenge and devour all that is dead and dying, returning it to the dust of the earth. Often perceived as pests or germs, reducer organisms are a misunderstood part of nature's food chain.

*They are, in essence, nature's clean-up crew—the greatest recyclers nature ever created.*

In essence, these "bugs" are not our enemy, and ecologically speaking, we could not exist without them. They complete nature's food chain cycle. Without them, dead plant and animal matter would build up, and important nutrients would remain locked inside. Our soils would become nutrient-poor and unable to support primary producers sufficiently, having a negative domino effect up the food chain.

## OUR BODY'S MICROBIOME

To understand nature's food chain and the inherent function of each species within the chain is to understand the great and ever-evolving cycles of life on Earth. Microbes are the oldest form of life on Earth. They were here long before we got here and will be here long after we leave. In fact, microbe fossils date back more than 3.5 billion years to a time when the Earth was covered with oceans, and hundreds of millions of years before dinosaurs roamed our planet. Earth, as we know it, wouldn't even exist without these tiny single-cell organisms, and neither would we.

Microbes are tiny single-cell organisms that are much too small to be seen by the human eye. And even though we can't see them without a high-powered microscope, they are everywhere! They are outside of us, and inside of us. They are in the air we breathe, the ground we walk upon, the water we drink, and the food we eat. We couldn't even digest our food or breathe without them.

Today, the microbiology scientific community calls the microbial world within us the microbiome. They discovered that the number of bacteria living within the average healthy adult outnumbers human cells ten to one. While the human body has approximately 36 trillion cells, our microbiome has approximately 39 trillion microbial cells, including bacteria, viruses, and fungi that live on and in us.

After researchers discovered that we live, move, and have our being within this ever-evolving microbial world, they went on a quest to better understand the workings of these communities that reside within us. Microbiome research has become one of the major health topics and studies of our time.

Their research now shows that disturbances within our body's microbiome might just be responsible for most of our modern-day diseases such as inflammatory bowel disease, digestive disorders, skin and gum disease, obesity, metabolic syndromes, and even HIV… just to name a few!

Margaret McFall Ngai of the University of Wisconsin, Madison, says…

> "This could be the basis of a whole new way of looking at disease. To understand how changes in normal bacterial populations affect or are affected by disease, we first must establish what normal is or if normal even exists."

For over a century now, medical science has waged war against these tiny single-cell organisms, using such things as antibiotics as their lethal weapons. But today, the warfare mentality (a mentality that can be viewed as collateral damage—wiping out the good with the bad) is changing as some microbiologists and scientists like Julie Segre, Ph.D., senior investigator at the National Human Genome Research Institute, have delved deeper into the trillions of microbes that call the human body home—collectively known as the microbiome.

Dr. Julie Segre said…

> "I would like to lose the language of warfare. It does a disservice to all the bacteria that have co-evolved with us and are maintaining the health of our bodies."

While the diversity of species that make up a microbiome is difficult for most scientists to fathom, I am grateful that some are finally becoming what I call "internal environmentalists"… those who study our internal terrain and the microbial environment in which these microbes live.

Now, for the first time ever, microbiologists are recognizing the importance of learning the best way to sustainably coexist with the trillions of microbial communities that live symbiotically within our internal environment.

Their benefits are numerous. They include…
- A highly efficient immune system
- Protection against the overgrowth of other microorganisms such as Candida/fungus, parasites, and pathogenic bacteria
- Protection against infection
- Proper digestion of food
- Absorption of nutrients

- Production of vitamins
- Elimination of toxins
- Detoxification of harmful chemicals

Prevention of allergies (microbes help to distinguish between harmful substances and healthy ones)

The key is to…

*Learn how to work with them and not against them!*

Natural feeding, which I will also refer to as natural eating—eating the way nature intended—for every species that exists within nature's food chain (including microbes), is the key to a healthy, sustainable life. When we have an in-depth understanding of the importance of "feeding" the right types of food into our body's internal environment, we'll completely demystify the word, disease.

Once again, the word disease means…

Dis ~ to move away from…
Ease ~the natural flow of life
(freedom from pain and suffering)

Dr. Will Bulsiewicz, board-certified gastroenterologist and best-selling author of Fiber Fueled: The Plant-Based Gut Health Program for Losing Weight, Restoring Your Health, and Optimizing Your Microbiome, has scientifically proven that when it comes to a healthy microbiome, a high-fiber, plant-based diet is everything! That means no meat, dairy, or ultra-processed foods—the foods that acidify and destroy the microbial balance within our body's internal environment.

Affectionately known as Dr. B, what he has discovered about our microbiome is rocking the scientific world. He and his team of scientists even found that during the time of COVID-19, those who had a healthy gut microbiome experienced little or no symptoms. He questioned the validity of wearing masks and social distancing by asking…

> "Was there really any merit to social distancing? And more importantly, how can you optimize the organ that's responsible for 70% of your immune system—your gut?"

We both agree that…

> *We can only experience a healthy, sustainable life by consuming the foods nature designed us to eat—PLANTS!*

In addition to eating a plant-based diet, a group of Japanese scientists spent over forty years in research and development using nanotechnology to develop products that would establish a healthy microbiome. They are known as the longevity company after uncovering the secret to living a long, healthy life—a symbiotic relationship with these tiny microbes! Interestingly, they do not classify these microbes as being "good or bad," but rather nature's balance between the two.

After investigating the "Centenarians," a group of people on the island of Okinawa who live over the age of 100 without degenerative diseases, they discovered the Centenarians' longevity health secret—

an intestinal bacterium that "speaks" to the brain and commands bodily functions to activate, repair, and protect.

In summary, when you live in harmony with nature and consume the foods nature designed you to eat, the microbial world within you will support you in having a long, healthy life while on Earth. On the other hand, if you consume the foods that are unnatural to your inherent design, the microbial world within you will perform their inherent job, which is to reduce your body back into the dust of the earth.

So stop playing victim and blaming a "bad bug" for any health challenge you may be experiencing. Microbes are a necessary part of nature's food chain, and the bottom line is…

*If you feed 'em… they're gonna' come!*

## — 5 —
# EAT RIGHT FOR YOUR ANATOMICAL TYPE

Let's face it; even if you're suffering from the onslaught of acidosis caused by internal acid rain, change is not always easy. Old habits that have been ingrained in us since childhood can be very strong and not so easy to break, especially when it comes to food. Most of us have a built-in need to "fit in," so whenever there's a family gathering or social event, it might be somewhat challenging to stick with your *New Earth Diet* lifestyle.

People may not understand the New You and may even think you've "lost a screw or two" because you no longer fit into their lifestyle. I know because it happened to me! That's when I had to become aware of my thoughts and feelings whenever "tribal" issues arose. Trust me, returning to the frugivore diet that you were designed to eat is not always easy. We all want to "fit in!"

The first thing required in shifting these deeply ingrained food habits and social indifferences is to simply watch the thoughts that run through your mind if they try to convince you that it's okay to eat this or that just this one time when you now know it isn't. Believe me, over these last 33 years, I've come face-to-face with every dietary roller coaster "hoop and loop" excuse you can possibly imagine.

Most of us will listen to the part of our mind that says...

*I'll start tomorrow!*

But for most, tomorrow never comes. Simply become aware of any thoughts or feelings that are behind your need to "fit in" with your "tribe" or any need of not wanting to feel something. Food can be a powerful "stuff it" mechanism, so be the observer; become aware.

So now, if you're ready, let's get started by examining every food and drink that veils and deadens the real you and which ones unveil and enliven the real you! You deserve to be all you came here to be!

After over 35 years of experiencing every health diet possible—all raw for seven years, macrobiotic for two years, vegetarian for seven years, vegan for 13 years—I can honestly attest that a frugivore diet has had the most positive effect on every aspect of my mind, body, emotions, and spirit.

Now that we've established that every biological species within nature's food chain (including microbes) has a natural way to "feed," let's take a deeper dive into where we, as humans, fit in. Inherently, we humans are a tropical species. We have lived in warm climates for most of our evolutionary history, which might explain why so many of us spend winter huddled under a blanket, clutching a hot water bottle, or spending wintry months in a warm climate.

Our species, Homo sapiens, have now spread to all parts of the world, but it's generally believed that we originated in Africa approximately 200,000 years ago. As such, we humans originally lived in a warmer, fruit-abundant climate, which made it easier for us to thrive within the confines of nature's food chain.

Within the hierarchy of the food chain, every species has an anatomical body type. As you will soon see, anatomically speaking, humans are not herbivores, omnivores, or carnivores, as some believe, but rather frugivores.

For some of you, frugivore may be a new term, but it's really very simple. Frugivores are a species whose preferred food is fruit, along with a small number of leafy greens, nuts, and seeds. Not only do frugivores feed on this diet, but they also thrive on it!

## HUMANS ARE FRUGIVORES BY NATURE'S DESIGN

While it is understandable for most vegans and vegetarians to think of humans as herbivores, as we have long been taught the importance of eating our "veggies," we are not. Our biological and anatomical design suggests that we are frugivores. While the notion of us being predominant fruit eaters may be an extremely radical viewpoint for most, it is imperative to be open to the possibility that we are, and that we were forced to physiologically adapt over millennia from our original tropical fruitarian diet—the diet that sustained a long, healthy life.

*Frugivores* are a group of primary consumers whose natural diet is to consume plant foods from trees and bushes that contain a very small amount of digestible cellulose found in fruits, seeds, nuts, and various leafy green vegetables.

*Herbivores*, on the other hand, consume grasses from the earth that contain a lot of cellulose. In essence, herbivores can digest large amounts of cellulose such as in leaves, stems, and roots, with the aid of symbiotic microorganisms; and frugivores do not.

As frugivores, if we found ourselves living in a tropical paradise without modern-day conveniences such as electricity, refrigeration, and grocery stores, our natural diet would be essentially the same as that of a primate such as a chimpanzee. That means we would be eating fresh, ripe, raw fruits (and some tender, leafy green vegetables, and shoots) right off the vine of a tree or a bush with the inclusion of small amounts of raw nuts and seeds.

After all, we are essentially 98 percent genetically, biologically, and anatomically identical to a chimpanzee.

Raw food advocate Victoria Boutenko, who is an expert on the raw, living food diet, thoroughly researched the diets of chimpanzees for her book Green for Life. She tells us that…

> "Chimpanzees are very similar to humans. Scientists at the Chimpanzee and Human Communication Institute at Washington Central University believe that chimpanzees should be categorized as people."

While we are obviously not completely identical to chimpanzees and did not evolve from apes as evolutionists may argue, we are close enough to consider our physiological similarities and how we relate particularly to food gathering, consumption, and digestion, and learn from them when they live in their natural habitat.

Anthropologist Dr. Katharine Milton, professor at the University of California, Berkeley, asserted that many characteristics of modern primates, including humans, derive from an early ancestor's practice of taking most of its food from a tropical canopy.

She stated…

> "Food eaten by humans today, especially those consumed in industrially advanced nations, bears little resemblance to the plant-based diets anthropoids (monkeys, apes, and humans) have favored since their emergence."

She also stated…

> "The widespread prevalence of diet-related health problems, particularly in highly industrialized nations, suggests that many humans are not eating in a manner compatible with their biology."

Our distant ancestors, whose gut proportions were virtually identical to our own, ate a wide variety of wild fruits, flowers, seeds, nuts, and green leaves, with only a small percentage of animal matter, probably less than two percent, and probably because of a rare need to survive. And, of course, none of this food was cooked until very late in our evolutionary development with the mastery of fire, around 500,000 years ago. A similarly late date can be established for weapon making, hunting, and a significant rise in meat consumption.

A very recent date, roughly 12,000 to 10,000 years ago, can be established for the period when the wide variety of plants previously consumed in the human diet became limited, for the most part, to a very narrow range of agricultural crops. And within this very narrow range of plants, actually monocultures in some areas, plants were almost immediately subjected to genetic modification through selective breeding, so that they now hardly even resemble the wild plants from which they were derived.

These are three relatively recent and quite radical departures from the raw, 98 percent frugivore or even herbivorous diet that had evolved over tens of millions of years along our ancestral line prior to their arrival. Our anatomy and physiology have a specifically corresponding diet, just like every other species of animal on this planet; and this diet was determined long before the adoption of fire, hunting, and agriculture. On the great evolutionary clock, there has simply not been enough time for the human body to adapt to these 'sudden' changes.

While we are technically only 1.6 percent different from chimpanzees and, surprisingly, closer to them in genetic structure than a dog is to a fox, a white-handed gibbon is to a white-cheeked crested gibbon, and an Indian elephant is to an African elephant, our diets are, indeed, extremely different today. This is especially true in the case of those consuming the Standard American Diet (SAD).

While there is a growing body of evidence emerging from researchers and scientists regarding the departure from our original diet and millennia of dietary adaptation, I believe that in the next several years we're going to see its connection to the diseases that have plagued humanity for a very long time.

Dr. Milton goes as far as to say…

> "Such findings lend support to the suspicion that many health problems common in technologically advanced nations may result, at least in part, from a mismatch between the diets we now eat and those to which our bodies became adapted over millions of years."

Consider that a chimpanzee's diet living in its natural habitat is predominantly fruit, comprising approximately 68 percent of its diet. The rest of a chimp's diet is the following: leaves 11 percent, seeds 7 percent, flowers 2 percent, bark 1 percent, pith 2 percent, insects 6 percent, and mammals 2 percent. Their diet is uncooked and unprocessed. Rarely do you ever see chimpanzees, bonobos (pygmy chimpanzees), and orangutans eating the flesh of an animal; and this would most likely be out of a need to survive. Other apes do not consume animals at all except in the form of insects as they are eating plant matter.

While it is true that I am advocating we consume a diet much like our closest relative, the chimpanzee, there are several differences…

> (1) On occasion, a chimpanzee might eat a few insects or an animal, but only if it's in a survival situation. Therefore, I would

never advocate the consumption of insects or animals.

(2) I believe that we are tropical beings by design; that we were never meant to live where fruit trees don't blossom and grow. So, if you live in Alaska, you may want to ask yourself, why? (Just teasing!), and...

(3) I also believe that our transition back to our original, natural way of eating needs to be slow and steady; that is, unless you are dealing with a major health issue like I was.

This is mostly because, through millennia of evolutionary adaptation, our diets and our environment have shifted and devolved in such a way that makes it necessary to make the transition slowly and wisely back into eating the diet that we were originally designed to eat. For some, it may even be difficult to imagine eating this type of diet since we are so very far and so long removed from it; but just being able to imagine what it might be, or might have been, could be a way of ushering in a new possibility and a new humanity!

## EXPLORING ANATOMICAL TYPES

Several hundred years ago, Carolus Linnaeus (1707-1778), the great taxonomist who established scientific methods for classifying plants and animals, recognized that humans were fruit eaters. He wrote...

> "Man's structure, internal and external, compared with that of the other animals, shows that fruit and succulent vegetables are his natural food."

We hold a unique place within the ecosystems of life. As primary consumers, we are frugivores, but no species' natural prey. No one hunts us. There are none above us in the food chain.

Francis Moore Lappé, a pioneer in identifying the environmental costs of the foods we eat, suggests that the meat-centered diet is unnatural to humankind.

She stated...

> "Traditionally the human diet has centered on plant foods, with animal foods playing a supplementary role. Our digestive and metabolic systems evolved over millions of years on such a diet. Only very recently have Americans, and people in some other industrial countries, begun to center their diets on meat. So, it is the meat-centered diet—and certainly the grain-fed-meat-centered diet—that is the fad."

There are many who agree with her. Cardiologist William C. Roberts, M.D., hails from the famed cattle state of Texas. He unequivocally believes that humans are not physiologically designed to eat meat and that when we kill animals to eat them, they end up killing us because their flesh, which contains cholesterol and saturated fat, was never intended for human consumption.

Unlike a meat-eating species, we lack both the physical characteristics of carnivores and the instinct that drives us to kill animals and devour their raw carcasses. We are physically and psychologically unable to rip animals' limbs from limb with our teeth.

Dr. Roberts stated…

> "I think the evidence is pretty clear. If you look at various physical characteristics of carnivores versus herbivores, it doesn't take a genius to see where humans line up."

Robert Morse, N.D., agrees with Dr. Roberts, except to clarify that humans are not just herbivorous plant eaters, but specifically frugivores, because of their anatomical design.

According to Dr. Bernard Jensen, a leading natural health physician and expert in juice therapy, said that Dr. Morse, the author of *The Detox Miracle Sourcebook*, is "one of the greatest healers of our time!"

Dr. Morse tells us…

> "Eat the foods that are biologically suited for your species!"

To illustrate the feeding habits natural to our anatomical design, Dr. Morse created the following chart comparing the typical anatomy and physiology of carnivores, omnivores, herbivores, and frugivores.

# ANATOMICAL TYPES CHART

| Carnivores such as cats, cheetahs, lions | Omnivores such as chickens, pigs, and dogs | Herbivores such as horses, cows, sheep, deer | Humans and primates such as apes, chimpanzees, and monkeys |
|---|---|---|---|
| **DIET** | | | |
| Mainly meats, some vegetables, grass, and herbs | Some meat, vegetables, fruits, roots, and some barks | Vegetables, herbs, and some roots, and barks | Mainly fruits, nuts, seeds, sweet vegetables, and herbs |
| **DIGESTIVE SYSTEM** | | | |
| Very rough tongue (for pulling and tearing) | Moderate to rough tongue | Moderately rough tongue | Smooth tongue, used mainly as a shovel |
| No salivary glands | Under-active salivary glands | Alkaline digestion starts with the salivary glands | Alkaline digestive energies start with the salivary glands |
| Stomach has a simple structure; small round sacks; strong gastric juices | Stomach has moderate gastric acids (HCL and pepsin) | Stomach is oblong, ringed, and the most complex (may have 4 or more pouches) | Stomach is oblong with 2 compartments |
| Small intestine is smooth and short | Small intestine is somewhat sacculated, enabling to eat vegetables | Small intestine is long and sacculated for extensive absorption | Small intestine is sacculated for extensive absorption |
| Liver is 50 percent larger that that of humans; very complex with fve distinct chambers; heavy bile flow for heavy gastric juices | Liver is complex and larger proportionately than that of humans | Liver is similar to human, though slightly larger in capacity | Liver is simple and average size, not large and complex like carnivores |
| **ELIMINATIVE SYSTEM** | | | |
| Colon is smooth, non-sacculated, with minimal ability for absorption | Colon is shorter than human colon, with minimal absorption | Colon is long and sacculated (ringed) for extensive absorption | Colon is sacculated for extensive absorption |
| GI tract is 3 times the length of the spine | GI tract is 10 times the length of the spine | GI tract is 30 times the length of the spine | GI tract is 12 times the length of the spine |

| EXTREMITIES | | | |
|---|---|---|---|
| Hands (upper front) with claws | Hands (upper front) are hoofs, claws, or paws | Hands (upper) are hoofs | Hands have fngers for picking, peeling and tearing |
| Feet (lower back) with clawsa | Feet (lower back) are hoofs, claws, or paws | Feet (lower) are hoofs | Feet have toes |
| Quadrupeds (walks on all fours) | Quadrupeds, except for birds, which walk on two legs | Quadrupeds | walks upright on two feet |
| INTEGUMENTARY SYSTEM | | | |
| Skin is 100 percent covered with hair | Skin is smooth, oily, and covered with hair or feathers | Skin has pores with hair covering the whole body | Skin has pores with minimal hair |
| Uses tongue to sweat, has sweat glands only in foot pads | Very minimal sweat glands; around snout (pigs) and (foot pads (dogs); none on birds | Millions of perspiration ducts for sweat glands | Millions of perspiration ducts for sweat glands |
| SKELETAL SYSTEM | | | |
| Incisor teeth in front, molars behind, large canine teeth for ripping | Tusk-like canine teeth or beaks | 24 teeth: 5 molars on each side of upper and lower jaw, and 8 incisors (cutting teeth) in the front of the jaw | 32 teeth: 4 incisors, 2 cuspids, 4 small molars, and 6 molars (no long canine or tusklike teeth) |
| Jaws are unidirectional, upand- down only | Jaws are multidirectional | Jaws are multidirectional, creating a grinding effect | Jaws are multidirectional |
| Tail | Tail | Tail | Some tail |
| URINARY SYSTEM | | | |
| Kidneys produce acid urine | Kidneys produce acid urine | Kidneys produce alkaline urine | Kidneys produce alkaline urine |

*From Robert Morse, N.D., The Detox Miracle Sourcebook (Prescott, AZ: Hohm Press, 2004).*

In essence, a cow was not designed to eat a fish or a chicken; it was designed to eat grass. Likewise, a human was not designed to eat a cow or grass; we were designed to eat fruit!

Since we are truly frugivores, our diet should consist of ripe raw fruits and vegetables, in particular, tender leafy greens, with the inclusion of small amounts of raw nuts and seeds. This is our perfect diet! And if you'll eat this way for about 90 days like I did, your life will change so drastically that you'll wonder where you've been all of your life!

Dr. Herbert Shelton, N.D., author of Superior Nutrition, tells us...

> "In fresh fruit, greens, vegetables, and nuts are all of the vitamins, minerals, proteins, and other substances the human body needs to bring it to a state of physical perfection and to maintain it in this state indefinitely!"

Always keep in mind that whenever any species goes against nature and eats food they were never designed to eat, they will eventually suffer devastating consequences. As an example, cows are grass-eaters. Yet in factory farms, cows are fed grains to fatten them up. As a result, these natural grass-eaters become very sick with severe acidosis and have to be kept alive with large doses of antibiotics until slaughter. Sadly, if they weren't slaughtered, they would die anyway from this forced, unnatural lifestyle. And while you may think that this is a horrific scenario (and it is), the truth is, our story is much the same.

Even though there's no one above us in the food chain, which means we're not going to be slaughtered for another animal's food (thank God!), we too have been eating foods that are biologically unsuited for our species. As a result, we have become very sick with severe acidosis and must treat our ills with large doses of antibiotics and various other drugs, just to stay alive! When this happens, the microbial world that resides within us becomes imbalanced, which in turn makes us subject to almost every disease known.

Thus, unnatural eating is the cause and natural eating is the cure!

Alkaline plant foods, foods from trees and bushes, are the foundational foods that fuel your body for life. These foods will alkalize you like nothing else.

Think about it—just as green plants of the earth fill our planet's atmosphere with lots of oxygen, a diet high in alkaline fruits and green plant foods will also fill your body's atmosphere with lots of oxygen. Thus, when you eat the diet that you were naturally designed to eat, you'll be alkalizing your way to wellness because you'll be eating the foods that support your natural alkaline design.

Then God said...

> "I give you every seed-bearing plant on the face of the whole earth and every tree that has fruit with seed in it. They will be yours for food."
>
> -Genesis 1:29

"And to all the beasts of the earth and all the birds in the sky and all the creatures that move along the ground—everything that has the breath of life in it—I give every green plant for food." And it was so.

-Genesis 1:30

OKAY, BUT!!! …

**Where Do I Get My Protein?**
One of the most common myths about a plant-based diet is that you will not get enough protein. The outdated belief that we need to consume meat for our daily requirements of protein has been completely invalidated. Although protein is certainly an essential nutrient that plays many key roles in the way our bodies function, we do not need huge quantities of it as some schools teach. In fact, fruits and vegetables contain more than adequate amounts of protein.

Think about how much protein is in mother's milk. Nature tells us that babies are best served with the modest level of 2 percent protein found in their mother's milk. Consider that babies grow more rapidly than at any other period throughout their entire lives. Their protein needs are, therefore, at a maximum. The biological reality is that we humans need very little protein in our diets.

However, most of us have been taught to believe by highly paid "under-the-table" lobbyists that animal protein is of a higher quality than plant protein and that good health is dependent upon getting enough animal protein in our diets. Fortunately, this is not the case. Our biological and anatomical needs for protein are as easily met by plant foods such as fruits and vegetables!

For your protein concerns, please consider the following lists:

## Amount of Protein in Fruit

**Avocado**: One medium size contains 4.02 grams of protein.
**Banana**: One medium size contains 1.29 grams of protein.
**Blackberries**: One cup contains 2 grams of protein.
**Blackcurrants**: One cup contains 1.57 grams of protein.
**Blueberries**: One cup contains 1.1 grams of protein.
**Boysenberries**: One cup contains 1.45 grams of protein.
**Cherimoya**: One cup contains 2.51 grams of protein.
**Cherries**: One cup with pits contains 1.46 grams of protein.
**Dates**: One cup contains 3.6 grams of protein.
**Gooseberries**: One cup contains 1.32 grams of protein.
**Grapefruit**: One cup contains 1.45 grams of protein.
**Grapes**: One cup contains 1.09 grams of protein.
**Guava**: One cup contains 4.21 grams of protein.
**Loganberries**: One cup contains 2.23 grams of protein.
**Lychee**: One cup contains 1.58 grams of protein.
**Mango**: One without peel contains 1.06 grams of protein.
**Mulberries**: One cup contains 2.02 grams of protein.
**Nectarine**: One cup contains 1.52 grams of protein.
**Orange**: One medium size contains 1.23 grams of protein.
**Passion fruit**: One cup contains 5.19 grams of protein.
**Peach**: One medium-size (with skin) contains 1.36 grams of protein.
**Plum**: One cup contains 1.15 grams of protein.
**Pomegranate**: One contains 4.71 grams of protein.
**Prickly Pear**: One cup contains 1.09 grams of protein.
**Raspberries**: One cup contains 1.48 grams of protein.
**Star fruit**: One cup contains 1.37 grams of protein.

**Tomato**: One medium size contains 1.08 grams of protein.
**Watermelon**: One medium wedge contains 1.74 grams of protein.

## Amount of Protein in Vegetables

**Alfalfa**, raw sprouted: One cup contains 1.32 grams of protein.
**Artichoke**: One medium size cooked without salt contains 3.47 grams of protein.
**Asparagus**: One-half cup (about 6 spears) cooked without salt contains 2.16 grams of protein.
**Beetroot**: One-half cup cooked without salt contains 1.43 grams of protein.
**Bok Choy**: One cup cooked without salt contains 2.65 grams of protein.
**Broccoli**: One cup cooked without salt contains 3.71 grams of protein.
**Brussels Sprouts**: One cup cooked without salt contains 3.98 grams of protein.
**Butternut squash**: One cup cooked without salt contains 1.84 grams of protein.
**Cauliflower**: One cup cooked without salt contains 2.28 grams of protein.
**Celeriac**: One cup cooked without salt contains 1.49 grams of protein.
**Celery**: One cup cooked without salt contains 1.25 grams of protein.
**Chinese broccoli**: One cup cooked without salt contains 1 gram of protein.
**Chinese cabbage**: One cup cooked without salt contains 1.78 grams of protein.
**Fennel**: One cup raw contains 1.08 grams of protein.
**French beans**: One cup cooked without salt contains 12.48 grams of protein.

**Kale**: One cup cooked without salt contains 2.47 grams of protein.
**Leek**: One cooked without salt contains 1 gram of protein.
**Mushroom**: One-half a cup contains 1.08 grams of protein.
**Okra**: One cup cooked without salt contains 3 grams of protein.
**Parsnip**: One cup cooked without salt contains 2.06 grams of protein.
**Potatoes**: One medium-size without salt contains 4.33 grams of protein.
**Pumpkin**: One cup cooked without salt contains 1.76 grams of protein.
**Spaghetti squash**: One cup cooked without salt contains 1.02 grams of protein.
**Squash, Summer**: One cup boiled without salt contains 1.87 grams of protein.
**Squash, Winter**: One cup baked without salt contains 1.82 grams of protein.
**Sweet Potatoes**: One medium baked contains 2.29 grams of protein.
**Swiss chard**: One cup cooked without salt contains 3.29 grams of protein.
**Turnip**: One cup boiled without salt contains 1.11 grams of protein.

*Data from USDA National Nutrient Database for Standard Reference, Release 25, and Dr. Decuypere's Nutrient Charts.*

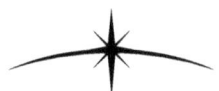

In summary, for all the intelligence we humans claim to have, what happened? Where did we go wrong? How did we shift into such a deep, hypnotic fallen state of dietary consciousness?

# — 6 —
# DIETARY DEVOLUTION

Sad, but true! Dietary devolution has not only made us sick, but it is also slowly and painfully sending us into an early grave. We have moved far away from a diet that supports our inherent anatomical design—a diet of fruits, green leafy vegetables, nuts, and seeds—a diet that sustains the life-sustaining microbial world within us. For most, unnatural eating has now become a socially accepted habitual way of living.

Dietary devolution accelerated when, long ago, we moved out of the tropics and shifted from a predominantly fruit-based alkaline diet as frugivores to a predominantly animal-based acidic diet as omnivores.

In 2009, Harvard Medical doctor, David L. Duffy, M.D., wrote…

> "A study in the Journal of Clinical Endocrinology and Metabolism finds that 'a diet that is high in (animal) protein and cereal grains is metabolized in a way that produces residue with an acidic pH. This may increase calcium excretion and weaken bones. I believe it may also inhibit the release of oxygen from the red blood cells to the body."

It has been well-documented that most degenerative diseases have increased in proportion to the number of acid ash-forming foods in our diet—foods that create a low-oxygen internal environment. This increase has occurred because we no longer eat the diet of our pre-agricultural ancestors—our original plant-based, alkaline ash-forming diet, abundant in life force energy.

The scant evidence that has survived from our remote past shows that modern-day humans slowly descended through three main dietary stages:

1. Fruitarian
2. Vegetarian/Herbivore
3. Omnivore/Carnivore

During the millions of years that we have inhabited the earth, our bodies have been forced to adapt to various environmental conditions and harmful pollutants to survive.

As our ancestors moved out of the tropics, they were forced to become hunter/gatherers; acid-producing meat and eggs were introduced. Along with agriculture and the domestication of animals, acid-producing dairy products, grains, and legumes were added to our diets. To add to an already acidic-based diet, we now have processed foods, junk foods, and fast foods. And as though all of that was not enough to send us into an "acidic state of inflammatory hell," we now have ultra-food processing methods that acidify both our bodies and our planet.

The epidemic basis of today's degenerative diseases can no longer be denied. The continuous downward acidic spiral of unnatural eating is at the root cause of most of our modern-day diseases. Simply put, a chronic buildup of acids in our tissues is what creates what I now call an ecological breakdown—an environmental crisis that destroys our body and our planet!

I say…

> *What we have long called disease is nothing more than a series of ecological breakdowns caused by burning the wrong types of food for fuel. Change the foods you're burning for fuel into your internal environment, and you'll not only change the course of your life but the course of the life of our planet as well!*

In the last century, dietary devolution has slid even further down the acidic scale—from an acidic omnivore/carnivore diet to the even more acidic chemivore diet, to the strongly acidic "junkivore" diet; and lastly, to the extremely acidic "drugivore" diet! These are new terms, admittedly, but they are meant to illustrate a point: not only have we moved far away from our original diet, but now many are consuming "foods" that aren't even foods!

Dietary devolution is characterized by the following:

### Vegetarian/Herbivore Diet
We shifted from our original, raw living food (pick, peel, and eat) frugivore diet and, instead, we began consuming a vegetarian/herbivore diet high in cultivated grasses, grains, and beans.

### Omnivore/Carnivore Diet
Then, we added animal flesh, eggs, and dairy products to our vegetarian/herbivore diet.

### Chemivore Diet
To make matters worse, we added petro-chemically, radioactively, and genetically contaminated genetically modified (GMO) plant foods to our omnivore/carnivore diet.

### Junkivore Diet
We are now consuming a diet high in chemivore-rich foods, foods that have been ultra-processed, denatured, and chemically altered; a diet that has sadly become the diet of the day.

### Drugivore Diet
And lastly, we are now forced to take handfuls of unnatural, life-altering synthetic drugs with breakfast, lunch, and dinner to alleviate our pain and suffering.

In writing about dietary devolution, I have a two-fold intention: (1) to unmask the grave problems we face and (2) to give you useful knowledge about how to navigate through our destructive modern-day food system so that you can help stop the devastating devolutionary slide—at least in your own and your family's life.

My motto is…

> *The actions we take today may not appear to make a difference in the world, but they have a rippling effect that has the power to significantly influence the greater whole.*

# DIETARY DEVOLUTION #1
## From Frugivore to Herbivore to Omnivore

As humans, we are a tropical species, designed to live in warm climates with trees of luscious ripe fruit to be picked, peeled, and eaten when hungry. Our anatomy still reflects that of other hominids, the great apes who are our closest relatives in the animal world. For millions of years, hominids have eaten primarily fruit. Anthropologist Alan Walker of Johns Hopkins University confirmed this through electron microscopy and other high-tech tools, from the examination of fossilized remains of early hominids.

Being natural fruit eaters, our earliest ancestors would have been guided by their sense of sight and smell to a sweet-tasting piece of fruit. They reached up to eat food from the trees or plucked berries from shrubs and vines.

Scientists tell us that Homo sapiens have walked the earth for less than 200,000 years, and during that time we have used tools to kill for meat. (This is especially true for those who wandered north or south to temperate and polar regions.) For this reason, there are those who view humans as natural omnivores rather than frugivores.

But it may be that archeologists have just scratched the surface of the multidimensional nature of our ancient history. There are myths and legends of great cities and high civilizations lost in the mists of time. There are records of astrophysical knowledge and technical feats, some of which we still cannot explain. The Hindu scriptures indicate that we had been on Earth four million years before the Great Deluge (the flood of Noah's time).

There are sources of knowledge other than the few fossil findings that have driven archaeological speculations about the human diet. Various threads of a fruitarian diet are woven throughout Greek historical accounts. For example, the ancient Greeks had very interesting things to say about the diet of those who came before them, and that was not so long ago.

Onomacritus of Athens (530-480 BC) said...

> "In the days before Lycurgus, each generation reached the age of 200 years."

A few centuries later, Plutarch (46-120 AD) observed that...

> "The ancient Greeks, before the time of Lycurgus, ate nothing but fruits."

Thus, we can deduce from these statements that the fruit-eaters were long-lived.

The indigenous people who lived in the region of the Aegean Sea before the ancient Greek civilization arose were known as Pelasgians. Hesiod (750-650 BC) said...

> "The Pelasgians and the peoples who came after them in Greece ate fruits of the virgin forests and blackberries from the fields."

A few centuries later, Philochorus (340-261 BC) said of the Pelasgians...

> "Their heroic spirit and their strong arms to destroy their foe were

formed of shiny red apples from the forest. Apples were their favorite food, and the speed of their feet never lessened. They raced against stags and won. They lived for hundreds of years in the world of Cronus, but as they grew old, their vast stature never diminished, even by a thumb's breadth. The dark luster of their black hair was never tainted by a single silver thread."

It may even be that in the beginning we did not eat food at all; that we lived on the light of God and the brilliant colors that imbued all of nature. I have had visions of such a time.

In the days before "The Flood," it was recorded that Methuselah, son of Enoch and the grandfather of Noah, lived to be 969 years of age. We cannot imagine this very long life today, so we discount it. But what if we were meant to live much longer, healthier, and more powerful lives—lives without sickness, disease, or pain?

Regardless of whether you believe in the literal occurrence of these events, we can know one thing for sure: sometimes we just don't know what we don't know. In other words, there is so much more of our past as a species that is not yet available to us. But what if we were truly designed to live much longer, healthier, and more productive lives? What if a state of perfect health is our natural state, rather than disease?

Even if we limit our vision of history to the conventional version, it seems clear that until very recently, most people lived according to their natural alkaline design, even among the hunter-gatherers who ate the meat of wild animals, but only on occasion. Findings among fossil records of early hunter-gatherers and studies of contemporary people living a hunter-gatherer lifestyle show a high ratio of living on raw, alkalizing plant foods versus acidic animal foods.

This diet creates a state of "mild, systemic metabolic Alkalosis"— alkaline values for blood, saliva, and urine. These findings by a group of clinical researchers from the University of California, among others, suggest that from an evolutionary perspective, an alkaline condition is the natural and optimal state of health for humans.

But today, a huge transformation has taken place in the human acid-alkaline metabolic environment. Due to the devolution of our diet, human beings are mostly living in a mild to severe state of acidosis. In doing so, we are going against our natural alkaline design, which is at the root cause of most of our diseases, shortening the days of our lives on Earth.

Mike Anderson, filmmaker and author of Eating, tells us...

> "Meat, dairy products, eggs, and fish were uncommon on the plates of working-class Americans. As animal foods became more affordable, Americans switched from their plant-based diets to animal-based diets. This triggered the biggest dietary devolution shift in human history and ushered in a new era of eating-related diseases. The biggest killer of humans in the history of life on this planet turns out to be the human appetite for animals."

The modern-day cultural omnivore diet consists of cooked meats of domesticated animals; animal products such as eggs and milk products (not ever part of a hunter-gatherer lifestyle); cooked grains and beans; vegetables, and an occasional salad or piece of fruit. In this scenario, meat, animal products, and grains are foremost, with a few side dishes of cooked, plant-derived mush.

Animal flesh and products, as well as grains, beans, and legumes, have replaced most of our original diet—the fruits of the tree and green plants of the vine. In the frugivore diet, fruit could be defined as encompassing not only the sweet fruits but fruits such as avocado, coconut, and the fruits of the vine, such as tomato, cucumber, and squash.

Mike Anderson summarizes the effects of an omnivore diet succinctly:

> "When people in other parts of the world abandon their traditional plant-based diets and start eating like Americans, they start dying like Americans. The pattern is not only obvious but is totally predictable. No matter where you look, when people adopt animal-based diets, heart disease and cancer suddenly become their biggest killers."

## DIETARY DEVOLUTION #2
## From Omnivore to Carnivore to Chemivore

Since the industrial revolution, eating from the top of the food chain has taken an even more disturbing turn. Sadly, carnivores, and in part, omnivores, feed from the top of the food chain chemical pot. Now, let's take a look to see how chemicals have permeated every part of our planet's environment as well as the environment of the human body, and how eating foods from the top of the food chain are hazardous to your health.

## How Chemicals Enter Our Food Chain

In recent years, Arctic waters, once relatively pristine, have become increasingly toxic. Chemicals from agricultural runoff, jet exhaust, industrial manufacturing, and the burning of fossil fuels have reached the farthest corners of the earth, carried by rivers, ocean currents, and winds.

Aquatic life in the Arctic feeds on plankton, which derives nutrients from ocean waters. In the process of collecting nutrients (a process called bio-accumulation), toxic pollutants also accumulate, making the pollutants much more concentrated in the cells of the plankton than in the surrounding water.

Because small fish consume vast amounts of plankton, these toxic chemicals concentrate in their flesh. This process, known as bio-magnification, repeats at each step of the food chain. Predators four to five links up the food chain are found to have accumulations of toxic chemicals in their tissues millions of times higher than that of the water they inhabit. The same principles apply to land animals.

Greenlanders, who traditionally eat almost entirely from the sea, tragically consume fish and other marine life that sit atop the food chain. Scientists are finding hundreds of hazardous synthetic compounds in the flesh of people inhabiting the Arctic tundra—at levels so extreme that the breast milk and tissues of some Greenlanders could be classified as hazardous waste.

The same principles of bio-accumulation and bio-magnification apply to land animals. The meat of farm animals, as well as wildlife, contains concentrated levels of toxins from contaminated feed and the toxic fields in which they graze. Today, eating meat is akin to taking your life into your own hands.

## Chemical Additives in Animal Feed

Toxic chemicals can make you fat. Toxins interfere with our metabolic systems and cause us to store fat. This may be in part because the body uses fat cells to store toxins it cannot easily eliminate. The body then resists breaking down fat cells in an attempt to protect itself from autointoxication.

Paula Baillie-Hamilton, M.D., reports that toxic chemicals such as organophosphates, carbamates, anti-thyroid drugs, steroids, antibiotics, and organochlorines are intentionally fed to livestock. These toxic classes of chemicals interfere with the weight-regulating hormones in cattle—and in humans. They are added to cattle feed in minute amounts—not enough to make the animals really ill, just fat!

Through bio-accumulation (from feed) and bio-magnification (in the case of animals fed on the carcasses of other animals, including feces and toxic chemicals), these toxins highly concentrate and end up on our plates as part of steak or hamburger.

The bottom line is...

> *Toxic chemicals can make you fat!*

So, if you want to lose weight, get off the chemical fatteners! If you must eat meat, eat the meat of organic, pasture-raised animals. Better yet, eat an organic, plant-based diet!

## Chemical Additives in Cold Cuts

Deli meats, lunch meats, cold cuts, bologna—whatever you call it—are processed meats. Hot dogs, Spam, and bacon also belong in this category. In addition to the environmental toxins and chemicals intentionally fed to animals, there are chemical additives mixed into processed meats. One commonly used additive in these processed meats is nitrates or nitrites. Nitrites artificially preserve the pink color of the meat so it won't turn gray and help prevent botulism.

During the processing of these meats, nitrites combine with amines (organic compounds of nitrogen) in the meat to form carcinogenic compounds. Unsurprisingly, studies of people who eat processed meats show a greater likelihood of contracting cancer.

## Chemical Stress Signals

The way we care for animals also affects our own health and well-being. The industrialization of animal husbandry, in which animals are treated merely as units of production, impacts us in profound ways. When a living being is subjected to high levels of physical, chemical, emotional, and mental stress and suffering, the body reflects that.

There are chemical stress signals: hormones are affected, metabolism is altered, and disease mechanisms are triggered.

When we eat the flesh of these animals, we consume the architecture of their suffering. Moreover, when we support factory farming by purchasing meat from markets, we participate in the ongoing suffering of animals. As Nelson Mandela said, "For to be free is not merely to cast off one's chains, but to live in a way that respects and enhances the freedom of others."

## Seafood from Toxic Oceans

Since the nuclear reactor meltdowns in Fukushima, Japan, radioactive contamination of seafood has become a real issue. Pacific Bluefin tuna spawn off the coast of Japan and swim across the ocean to school in the waters along the coast of California and Baja California, Mexico. In May 2012, a report in the Huffington Post revealed that levels of radioactive cesium in these great fish were ten times higher than usual.

Sea vegetables (aka seaweeds), like fish, have also come under suspicion of radioactive contamination. Since the Fukushima nuclear power plant meltdowns in Japan, reports have surfaced of radiation-contaminated sea vegetables being sold in the United States.

Michael Collins, writing for EnviroReporter on April 20, 2012, reports…

> "On April 13, 2012, EnviroReporter.com tested Nori seaweed from Japan bought in a West Los Angeles store, the same one where this reporter bought the identical item eight months ago soon after the Fukushima Daiichi meltdowns began in Japan. The trendy and 'organic' delicacy, popular with LA hipsters, was 94.7 percent above normal, 17.6 percent of that additional ionization indicative of alpha radiation which can be 60 to 1,000 times more dangerous than beta and gamma radiation."

He also notes that it is possible for the Japanese to export radiation-contaminated food products that do not even meet their standards to the United States—"standards up to dozens of times laxer for the kinds of radioactive particles spewing out of the nuclear plants in Fukushima."

It has become important to check the source of sea vegetables. Not all sea vegetables from Japan are contaminated, but some may be. For now, I would recommend buying from highly reputable sources like Maine Coast Sea Vegetables. Uncontaminated sea vegetables are a great source of iodine and help detoxify radioactive substances from the body.

**The Dangers of Mercury Toxicity**

Yet another factor to consider in eating fish is mercury toxicity. Have you ever wondered how mercury ends up in fish? Look to the coal industry, as coal contains some mercury. When coal is burned in power plants for electricity, that mercury goes out of the stack. It eventually falls onto the earth, or into the oceans, in the rain. It is taken up along with nutrients from the sea in the growth of plankton. Small fish feed on the plankton and are eaten by larger fish, which are eaten by yet larger fish, which are then eaten by people. What goes around comes around, as they say. Here is a simple illustration of how mercury toxicity works:

Some people believe that eating farm-raised fish is a healthy choice, and there's no reason it couldn't be. But, unfortunately, in our industrialized world, farm-raised fish are much more contaminated than the already extremely contaminated wild fish.

Studies in 2004 and 2005 showed farm-raised salmon with higher levels of mercury and ten or eleven times higher levels of carcinogens than wild-caught fish. To complicate matters, much of the fish that is labeled "wild-caught" is actually farm-raised, due to loopholes in the law and lax enforcement by the USDA.

But if you still want to include fish in your diet, you may want to consider fish that are lower on the food chain and wild-caught: mackerel, sardines, herring, oysters, and shrimp, for instance. Remove the skin. Realize though that when you fish and eat species in which mercury and other toxins are less concentrated, we are also removing the food sources of larger, longer-lived fish like tuna, cod, and snapper, thereby causing breakdowns in marine ecosystems. It is a no-win situation. Ending pollution, cleaning up the oceans, and switching to a plant-based diet is the only real answer.

**Drugged Cows and Pasteurized Dairy Products**
First, there are the chemical contaminants like drugs, pesticide-laced feed, and growth hormones that enter milk from industrial farming practices. In addition, pasteurization and homogenization both profoundly alter the chemical structure of milk, making it a food unfit for human consumption.

The common practice of pasteurization involves heating milk to 145°F for 30 minutes or 163°F for fifteen seconds (called flash pasteurization). The use of heat to destroy objectionable bacteria also destroys enzymes, beneficial bacteria, and nutrients.

Homogenization is a process whereby milk is pushed through a fine filter at pressures of 4,000 pounds per square inch. The structure of the milk proteins is changed—degraded, actually. Homogenization is used to create uniformity of flavor and fat content in large batches of milk. It keeps the cream from separating and rising to the top.

The health dangers of pasteurized and homogenized milk are:

- Processing the milk kills beneficial bacteria, leaving large batches of milk susceptible to environmental contamination by pathogenic bacteria, and large outbreaks of illness are more common than we realize.
- Processing the milk destroys enzymes and vitamins—especially C, B6, and B12, and alters milk proteins, making them less digestible.
- Calcium in the milk is less available, due to altered milk fats and the destruction of enzymes.
- May contain assorted drugs and antibiotics, pesticides from treated grains, bacteria from infected animals, and genetically engineered growth hormones (rBST or rBGH).
- Associated with diminished resistance to disease, increased risk of bone fractures, and high cholesterol.
- Known for its role in triggering health problems such as allergies, nasal congestion, constipation, increased tooth decay, anemia, arthritis, osteoporosis, atherosclerosis, leukemia, prostate cancer, ovarian cancer, nephrosis, and heart disease.
- Can trigger autoimmune diseases such as diabetes, Lou Gehrig's disease, or multiple sclerosis.
- Associated with infant and childhood illnesses such as ear infections, strep infections, colic, iron-deficiency anemia, asthma, growth problems, and antisocial behavior.

Most people believe that milk stamped with an organic certification assures a higher standard. Unfortunately, this is not always true. Organic milk in grocery stores is mostly ultra-pasteurized. Ultra-pasteurization does even more damage to milk than the usual process of pasteurization. The plastic or plastic-lined packaging also leaches various endocrine-disrupting compounds into the milk. Thus, organic, ultra-pasteurized milk falls squarely into the chemivore level of dietary devolution.

Milk found on grocery-store shelves today is very different from what our farming ancestors drank. Raw milk that comes from cows grazing on green pastures is a slightly alkaline food. This is because cows eat grass, which is highly alkaline. But it is high in fat, so why get your chlorophyll secondhand?

Did you know that milk comes in two varieties? They are known as A1 and A2. A1 and A2 refer to a minor difference in the position of an amino acid in beta casein, the protein in milk. Until about five thousand years ago, there was only one type of milk, what we call A2. Then, a genetic mutation occurred in some cattle, and they began to produce A1 milk. Some cows today still produce A2 milk, but most of the dairy cows in the United States are producers of A1 milk. Though the genetic difference is very slight, the effects are significant.

A New Zealand study called the Fonterra study found that neurological and mental disorders could be induced or aggravated by drinking A1 milk. There's also some evidence showing associations between the A1 casein in milk and increased risk of heart disease and diabetes. Drinking A2 milk did not have the same disease-causing effects.

Chemical toxins, including pesticides, are bio-accumulated and bio-magnified in dairy products too, especially in the fatty portion of the milk—the cream and the butter made from that cream.

This occurs mostly because most modern industrial chemicals, including pesticides and drugs, are derived from petroleum (oil)! In pumping oil from underground veins, one could say that we are extracting the "fat of the land." Chemicals created from this fat of the land are fat-soluble (requiring fats for digestion and absorption rather than water) and, therefore, end up in the fatty portions of animal products and in our fatty tissues.

## Produce From Toxic Chemical-Laden Fields
Our agriculture and food supply are now characterized by...

- Intensive, widespread irrigation on marginal, depleted soils.
- Chemically intensive cropping.
- Genetic engineering of seed.
- Centralization of ownership and distribution in a few hands.
- Long shipping distances.
- Chemical additives, preservatives, and irradiation.
- Poor flavor and lower levels of nutrients.

Agriculture as we know it today is not sustainable. It is consumer agriculture—consuming resources without replenishing them. As with the extraction of oil in the fossil fuel industry, resources of land and water are being used up at an incredible rate.

Billions of pounds of chemicals are applied to the land in an attempt to prop up soil fertility and reduce crop destruction from pests. The result is the destruction of the microbial life of the soil and beneficial insects, including bees and butterflies.

Toxic pesticides banned for use here are still used on crops in various foreign countries. For example, many fruits and vegetables are imported from Mexico, especially in the wintertime. Sadly, only a small percentage of the billions of pounds of food imported into the United States are inspected for pesticide residues.

Pesticide and fungicide residues and waxes are very difficult to wash off fruits and vegetables, and peeling off the skin does not keep us safe either, as chemical residues are often absorbed into the flesh of the produce. Then, there are insecticides that are part of the plant's genetic structure, like Bt-toxins in Monsanto's (one of America's leading multinational chemical conglomerates) genetically modified sweet corn. Can't wash those off!

There is a growing body of research on petroleum-based chemicals and pesticides. Pesticides have been shown to cause significant weakening effects on the nervous system and immune system. Illnesses identified in the medical research include adult and child cancers, numerous neurological disorders, immune system weakening, autoimmune disorders, asthma, allergies, infertility, miscarriage, and child behavior disorders, including learning disabilities, mental retardation, hyperactivity, and attention deficit disorders (ADD). These are just some of the effects of toxic load and chronic acidosis.

Identifying a specific chemical (or mycotoxin, see below) as the original cause of health disorders in the general population is difficult and often overlooked, as it typically requires years of exposure for the body's inherent defenses to weaken sufficiently to result in observable health problems. Also, many of our illnesses result from a combination of petroleum-based chemicals working in tandem, making specific identification even more difficult.

Paula Baillie-Hamilton, M.D., author of *The Body Restoration Plan*, says that the ever-increasing role of petroleum as a basis of our society throughout the last century parallels the ever-increasing role of acidosis as a basis of the diseases from which we suffer.

**Chemicals and Toxic Mycotoxins**
Like invasive forms of Candida, other fungi can exude poisonous substances called mycotoxins. Mycotoxins are toxic secondary metabolites produced by fungi and are capable of causing disease and death in both humans and animals. The term 'mycotoxin' usually refers to toxic chemical products produced by fungi that readily colonize crops.

Chemical-laden, toxic fields have been shown to spawn mycotoxins. Higher levels of mycotoxins have been reported in grains grown under high-yield, chemically intensive farming systems. A study by The Organic Center on matched pairs of foods found that mycotoxins were a more serious issue in conventionally grown foods—twice as often at levels twice as high. Are conventionally farmed fields moldier?

Synthetic nitrogen fertilizer stimulates higher levels of fungal growth. When fertilizer-stimulated fungal populations come under stress from bad weather or other environmental difficulties, they produce mycotoxins as part of their survival response.

Then, there's the big problem. Monsanto's favorite organophosphate herbicide, and the most widely used herbicide in the world, Round-up (common name glyphosate), can accumulate and persist in the soil for years. Our extensive use of Round-up over the last thirty years has destroyed the balance of microbes in our agricultural soils, locking up soil nutrients, meaning they are no longer available to plants. Microbes are to the soil what friendly bacteria are to your intestinal tract.

Round-up not only destroys protective bacteria in the soil but also promotes more aggressive and virulent pathogens—particularly the family of fungi known as Fusarium. Applications of fungicide to control fungal eruptions caused by Round-up can trigger further mycotoxin outbreaks in field crops. This is because applying fungicide doesn't instantly kill all of the fungus in a field. The fungus that doesn't die immediately becomes highly stressed, and its defense mechanisms move into high gear with an explosion of mycotoxins.

Dr. Don Huber, Professor Emeritus of Plant Pathology at Purdue University, remarked...

> "What we have with glyphosate is the most abused chemical we have ever had in the history of man."

When applied to crops, Round-up becomes systemic throughout the plant, so it cannot be washed off. Once you eat this plant or its seed, the glyphosate ends up in your gut, where it can decimate your beneficial bacteria, just as it does the beneficial microbes in the soil. This is true for all crops grown with Round-up, not just "Round-Up Ready" GMOs.

The genus Fusarium creates more than a dozen known mycotoxins, which affect the nervous and endocrine systems. Dr. Don Huber also notes...

> "You look at Alzheimer's, thyroid problems, autism, Parkinson's—any of those diseases that have a tie with either the endocrine system or nutrient availability. We're going to see those [diseases] increase."

Round-up and glyphosate, marketed under various names, produce a double whammy: (1) the direct effect of the chemical residue in our intestinal tract, which destroys the balance of microorganisms and reduces nutrient bioavailability, and (2) the Round-up-stimulated fungal mycotoxins and their various deadly systemic effects.

In 2007, the USDA asked for permission to stop recording how much glyphosate we use. Dr. Huber remarks...

> "It was going up so rapidly that it was embarrassing, I think, for anybody to realize how much of this organic phosphate was being put out... We're seeing the effect on organisms in the intestinal tract just from the residue in the food and feeds."

You could say, perhaps, that mycotoxins are the "stress hormones" of the soil kingdom. Exceedingly low concentrations of mycotoxins (parts per billion) can have devastating effects when ingested. They are particularly known for disrupting the endocrine system, which makes sense since our endocrine system is involved in the management of stress and trauma. By consuming the chemical stress signals of the soil, we essentially take them upon ourselves. We can expect that mycotoxins will have various effects in the body, similar to our own chemical stress signals.

Mycotoxins are not only a problem in the field but can also arise from mold growth in the storage of grains and other foods. Fungal infestations and their poisonous excretions are also a growing problem in our homes and businesses.

Pathological fungi and molds can gain a greater foothold in deoxygenated areas. To maintain a mold-free body, keep your friendly intestinal populations strong and happy in an alkaline and oxygen-rich environment, fed by fresh, organic fruits and vegetables!

## The Dangers of Irradiated Foods

One of the latest additions to chemical devolution is the exposure of our food to radioactivity to extend its shipping or shelf life. Foods being irradiated include meats, grains, herbs, and produce. Irradiated food is generally bombarded with radiation five thousand to one million times greater than a chest x-ray.

The results of this exposure in foods include:
- Creation of free radicals.
- Damage to nutrients (may lose up to 80 percent of vitamins).
- Damage to enzymes.
- Creation of unique radiolytic (chemical breakdown using radiation) products. (Some of these chemical byproducts of irradiation are known toxins, while others are unique to irradiated foods, their effects as yet undocumented.)
- Tendency of fat to become rancid.
- Damage to the DNA of the living cells of the food.
- Trace amounts of lingering radioactivity.

Raw foods that have been irradiated look just like fresh foods, but nutritionally they are more like cooked foods, with decreased vitamins and enzymes. Still, the FDA allows these foods to be labeled fresh.

Treating solid foods with radiation provides an effect similar to the heat pasteurization of liquids, such as milk. While irradiation is a fundamentally different process, some ironically use the term "cold pasteurization" to describe the irradiation of foods.

It is hard to say how widespread irradiation is, but many restaurants and most fast-food outlets use irradiated foods. Many items in the grocery store include irradiated ingredients. If an entire product is irradiated, the symbol for international irradiation, the radura, should be shown on the product's package. However, when irradiated food is used as an ingredient in a product, the symbol is not required.

## Stop the GMO Madness!

GMO, short for "genetically modified organisms," are engineered to produce their own pesticides or survive direct application of pesticides. From GMO crops doused with pesticides to the patented seeds that farmers must buy and can't reuse, GMOs cause concern from farm to table. GMO foods and pesticides have a toxic relationship that's playing out in your grocery store and probably your kitchen.

Genetic engineering involves taking genes from one strain of a plant, animal, or microorganism and inserting them into another with the goal of introducing desired characteristics, such as increasing a plant's resistance to insects or enhancing the sweetness of a fruit. The practice is undertaken in part for economic reasons. If genetically modified plants become more resistant to harmful microbes and insects, yields improve.

However, bits of genetic material from organisms that have never been a part of the human food supply are changing the fundamental nature of the food we eat. Thus, when a plant's genes are manipulated, the result is no longer a plant due to animal, fungus, and mutated genes mixed into it. It is a genetically modified organism (GMO).

Arpad Pusztai, one of the first scientists to raise concerns about the safety of genetically modified foods, stated...

> "Gene insertion is a major problem. You cannot direct where the splicing of the genetic construct will happen. It is well known that when you insert a genetic construct into the DNA network of a plant, you create changes in that network. As a result, you will get changes in the functionality of the plant's own genes. They may become more active or silent. The effects will be unpredictable and uncontrollable. It can sometimes cause irreparable damage to the genome. This is called insertional mutagenesis."

In other words, the practice of genetic modification creates unpredictable, uncontrollable, and sometimes irreparable damage to the genome. Biotech scientists are experimenting with delicate yet powerful forces of nature without full knowledge of the widespread repercussions. Without long-term testing, how could they say that these foods are safe?

Here's an example that illustrates the politics of GMOs:

> Research published in the International Journal of Biological Sciences (2009) showed that three varieties of genetically modified corn caused organ damage in rats. (There were no human

studies.) All three varieties had been approved by numerous food safety authorities and are widely available in the United States, Europe, and elsewhere.

These were all Monsanto varieties. As mentioned earlier, Monsanto is one of the largest (multiple-billion-dollar) biotechnology corporations in the world, developing and patenting genetically engineered seeds. The data used by Monsanto for the approval of these GMO varieties is the same raw data that independent researchers studied to make the organ-damage link. They found serious mistakes in Monsanto's analysis of the data.

And in case you are wondering, these GMO varieties are still on the market, along with several new varieties of GMO corn, including sweet corn. To ensure that you are not purchasing any type of produce or prepackaged food or snack product (such as popcorn) that was grown with a GMO seed, be sure to look for the Non-GMO Project Verified seal.

**Unraveling the Genetic Strand**
Pesticides and other toxins generally diminish over time when left in the environment. Even if it takes a long time, eventually, they break down into less harmful compounds. Unlike most toxins, when GMOs are released into the environment, they do not revert to their original nature over time. Instead, they have the effect of unraveling and corrupting the genetic integrity of all life, especially those families of life to which they are closely related.

Experience has shown that a small release from a field of GMO canola plants, for instance, will increase its presence in nearby non-

GMO canola fields each following season. The GMO canola will also cross-pollinate with nearby weeds of similar botanical families. When these weeds regrow from seed the next season, they are now also genetically modified.

Even small amounts of GMO contamination will take over large areas and families of plants over time, with no end in sight.

Irradiation and genetic modification have in common the introduction of "strange chemistry," both known and unknown, through changes in the deep molecular structure of the seed, plant, fruit, meat, eggs, or milk. They wreak havoc by changing the original nature of our food from within.

The blueprint of these species is not being changed by natural evolution, or even by selective breeding, but by the bombardment of the DNA by a group of people who are playing God. When man thinks that he knows better than the Creator and the creation itself, it means trouble. We have no idea what this adulteration will lead to. Ultimately, in our callous willingness to manipulate other forms of life, we may be putting our own "seed"—the seeds of future generations—at risk.

Michael Pollan, a leading writer on food policy, said in a recent interview on GMO technology...

> "The real benefit of GM [Genetic Modification] to these companies is really the ability to control the genetic resources on which humankind depends...It represents a whole new level of corporate control over our food supply—a handful of companies are owning the seeds, controlling the farmers, and controlling our choices."

## Stop Eating Fake Fat

Junk-food manufacturers have been keenly aware of the criticism that their products contribute to obesity. To counter this, they created fake, zero-calorie sweeteners and fake fat as alternatives. While it's wise to avoid excessive fat—especially since many toxic chemicals in our food are stored in the fatty tissues of animals and fish, in cream and butter, and in vegetable oils—it's just as important to avoid fake fats. Ironically, like fake sweeteners, fake fats can also contribute to weight gain.

In 1996, the FDA approved Olestra, marketed under the brand name Olean, as a fat substitute in snack foods. Though its popularity has fluctuated, it is still used in some low-fat or fat-free snacks.

Olestra is a type of fat that is indigestible, meaning it passes through the body without being absorbed. However, it can also carry away essential fat-soluble nutrients, including carotenoids like lutein, beta-carotene, and lycopene, which are vital antioxidants. Olestra also depletes the body of fat-soluble vitamins A, D, E, and K.

Studies have highlighted Olestra's impact on nutrient depletion. For example, consuming the equivalent of sixteen Olestra-based, fat-free Pringles chips daily for two weeks reduced lutein levels in the blood by 20 percent. Similarly, consuming six chips a day for four weeks decreased blood lycopene levels by 40 percent.

Furthermore, Olestra can lead to weight gain. A 2011 study published in Behavioral Neuroscience found that rats fed a high-fat diet supplemented with fat-free Pringles gained more weight than those fed regular, high-fat Pringles. Researchers theorized that when the body expects a high-calorie intake based on sensory signals but doesn't receive the anticipated calories, it disrupts the body's energy regulation, leading to weight gain.

It's challenging to determine how many other toxic chemicals might be hidden under terms like "natural" and "artificial flavors." For instance, salt might come with dextrose, potassium iodine, and aluminum additives, while bread and processed cheeses could contain aluminum additives as well.

Junkivores—those who eat a diet dominated by junk food—are essentially meat-eating chemivores who have devolved into consuming a degraded diet. Unfortunately, many vegetarians and even some vegans have also fallen into the trap of a denatured, acidic, junkivore diet. The Urban Dictionary defines a "junkitarian" as someone who technically avoids meat but still consumes mostly junk food.

This is why some vegetarians I've consulted with are as acidic and sick as those who eat processed or otherwise unhealthy meats. In short, they are "junkitarians" rather than true vegetarians. A true vegetarian should be someone who consumes vegetation (whole plant foods), not someone who includes processed foods like potato chips in their diet, even if they come from health food stores and carry an organic label.

Ultimately, the real cost of a junkivore diet will likely include medical interventions such as drugs, surgeries, and other conventional disease management methods. In fact, medical bills now account for more than 60 percent of all bankruptcy filings in the United States.

# DIETARY DEVOLUTION #3
## From Chemivore to Junkivore to Drugivore

The junkivore diet is already nearly drug-like, driven more by chemical addiction than by a need for nourishment. In the final stage of dietary devolution, drugs begin to replace missing nutrients as the foundation for bodily functions, mental health, and immunity.

Sadly, we live in a world with a war-like mentality—whether it's the war against "bugs" or diseases like cancer. Billions of dollars are spent each year on research for cures, but is it truly curative? Every winter, we're encouraged to get a flu shot to fend off the season's "bugs," without ever being told that avoiding overindulgence during the holidays or fasting for a few days could help prevent the flu by eliminating accumulated, undigested waste that feeds those bugs.

Like using pesticides on a sick plant to kill the "bugs," drugs like antibiotics are used to kill invaders—often to the detriment of the ecological balance of our inner microbial world. Drugs, including flu shots, immunizations, and antibiotics, can have a profoundly debilitating effect on the trillions of microorganisms that populate our internal environment. You could say that within us, on a microscopic level, there is a landscape—an internal terrain—as remarkable as that of the Earth, or even the universe, populated by beneficial and harmful inhabitants.

Consider this astounding fact...

> There are at least ten times as many bacteria in the human body as there are cells.

Even the mitochondria—the power plants of our cells—may have evolved from a symbiotic relationship with free-living bacteria. Unfortunately, drugs wipe out our microbial populations and, worse yet, trigger the mutation of extremely harmful superbugs.

Another consideration is the side effects of drugs. Have you ever listened to the side effects listed in TV commercials? They're pretty scary, yet people still take these drugs!

In 1982, Dr. Bernard Jensen wrote:

> "The United States Department of Health, Education and Welfare's Task Force on Drug Prescriptions has reported that physicians tend to over-prescribe medicines, both in quantity and variety, for the same illness. About 300,000 people in this country are hospitalized each year for severe adverse drug reactions. Approximately 18,000 die annually from side effects of [prescription] drugs. Many patients become ill from medications without getting any benefit from them."

Just ten years later, those figures had skyrocketed: More than 1.8 million Americans suffered serious, toxic side effects from medical drugs and had to be hospitalized. By 1996, over two million Americans per year were hospitalized due to toxic effects of medications, and nearly 700,000 Americans died annually from secondary side effects of medications. Pharmaceutical drugs are more dangerous than most people realize.

Ultimately, drugs impact our internal landscape by...

- Creating other diseases that they call "side effects."
- Waging war on the complex web of living organisms and organic structures that constitute our metabolism.
- Decreasing the biodiversity of bacteria in the intestinal tract.
- Destroying the acid/alkaline balance, oxygenation, and hydration of the internal landscape.
- Polluting our fluid systems, leading to further degeneration of the nervous system and organs.
- Reducing sexual function and fertility.
- Directly poisoning and killing us. Prescription drugs are one of the leading causes of death in the U.S.
- Chronically weakening our lives and those of animals through water supplies contaminated by trace amounts of numerous drugs.
- Triggering the mutation of destructive superbugs, aggressive reducer organisms immune to our medical weapons.

Drugs are part of a medical industry that no longer cures diseases but rather manipulates and manages them. Mainstream medicine isn't about restoring the integrity of our internal landscape (as in the days of Hippocrates); it's about annihilating microbes through chemical warfare. This is why one drug often leads to another, and then another, as ecological breakdowns are accelerated until, by the age of 70, you're taking a handful of drugs with every meal, only to eventually die a very painful, disease-ridden death.

A powerful research paper titled Disease in Human Evolution (1996) describes how historical changes in lifestyle and landscape created conditions for new diseases and epidemics within human populations.

The most significant changes occurred with the advent of "better living through chemistry!" As cities sprang up, they created conditions for infectious epidemics and widespread malnutrition and diseases.

In the last century, among populations in developed and developing nations, infectious diseases declined while chronic degenerative diseases rose dramatically. Now, we are on the cusp of a third epidemiological transition—a reemergence of antibiotic-resistant "superbugs" capable of spreading globally.

Sadly, we now live in a world with a degraded environment, both inside and out. We are vulnerable to new, drug-resistant varieties of infectious disease and previously unknown infectious diseases. We are, in effect, taking infectious disease to a new level.

In previous centuries, epidemic infectious diseases were local or regional in nature. Now, with air travel, a new viral or bacterial infection can spread worldwide within days. The following conditions, which could be termed cultural disease vectors, have the potential to breed infectious disease across our world and redefine how we live—or even whether we live...

- The crossing of pathogens between species (as seen in mad-cow disease, for example).
- The destruction and pollution of natural ecosystems.
- The problems of dense population centers.
- Elevated levels of nuclear radiation and the proliferation of nuclear arms.
- The spreading of GMO seeds from farm to farm.

- Paula Baillie-Hamilton's macrobiotic adaptation (drug and pesticide resistance).
- The morphing of microbiota into pathological forms within the degraded environment of our internal landscape.

While this chapter offers a grand overview of the current state of our food affairs, perhaps we could echo the words of Charles Dickens from A Tale of Two Cities:...

> "It was the best of times, it was the worst of times, it was the age of wisdom, it was the age of foolishness, it was the epoch of belief, it was the epoch of incredulity, it was the season of Light, it was the season of Darkness, it was the spring of hope, it was the winter of despair, we had everything before us, we had nothing before us, we were all going direct to heaven, we were all going direct the other way—in short, the period was so far like the present period, that some of its noisiest authorities insisted on its being received, for good or for evil, in the superlative degree of comparison only."

For too long, we have operated from a mentality of domination—over one another, other species of life, and all of nature. But now, we've reached a point where we can break free from our fallen nature and return to our original spiritual nature, imbued with a consciousness that remembers paradise.

The only question that remains is...

*Are you ready to shift with me?*

# PART TWO
*The Return*

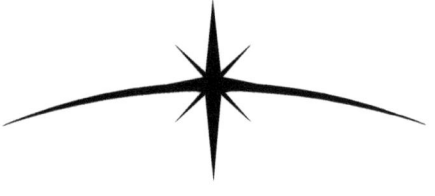

— 7 —

# ENLIGHTEN YOURSELF WITH NATURE'S FOUR "FUEL" GROUPS

Food isn't just a delectable substance that you put in your mouth, chew, and swallow. It's any micro or macro element that provides every cell in your body with the nutrients needed for energy and growth. While achieving perfect health and wellbeing does involve consuming plant foods grown in organic, nutrient-rich soil, it's crucial to remember that these foods are nurtured by more than just the earth—they require air, sunlight (fire), and water as well. Therefore, your physical body also needs constant support from these elemental forces.

The four elemental forces—earth, air, fire, and water—are not only the building blocks of your physical body but they are also the very foundation of the physical universe and the world of matter.

In classical Greek science and medicine, the four-elemental composition of a substance, in varying proportions, determines its nature, attributes, properties, and actions…

- **Earth**: Solid state – The plant foods we eat.
- **Air**: Gaseous state – The air we breathe.
- **Fire**: Incandescent state – The sunlight we absorb.
- **Water**: Liquid state – The water we drink.

To achieve perfect health, we must align ourselves with these dynamic four elements and fuel our bodies with the plants we eat, the air we breathe, the sunlight we absorb, and the water we drink. Instead of counting fats, carbohydrates, or protein as the foundation of the food pyramid, consider a new approach that I call... Nature's Four Fuel Groups!

# NATURE'S FOUR FUEL GROUPS
## Earth – Air – Fire – Water

These dynamic four—earth, air, fire, and water—do not fit within the confines of a man-made food group pyramid. Instead, they form the very structure of your physical body and work together in a synergistic field of movement, each one of equal importance.

Because these powerful elements create the very structure of your physical body, they are the "four fuel groups" of the *New Earth Diet*. By following their basic principles, you can cultivate a state of health and wellbeing that far surpasses the scope of most imaginations.

Remember, no matter what SOS signal your body may be sending you or whatever disease label you may have been given, if you work with these four dynamic forces of nature and not against them, you will not only turn your body's SOS signal around, but you will also begin the journey of ENLIGHTENING YOURSELF!

In essence, you'll begin the transformational journey of remembering who and what you truly are!

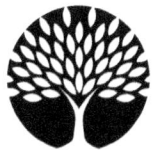

# EARTH
## Eat to Enlighten Yourself

To prepare our physical bodies for the shift of the ages—from a descended state of consciousness, often referred to as The Fall, to an ascended state of consciousness that I call The Return—it is crucial to begin by rethinking everything we've been taught about food, especially regarding the right diet for humans.

To make this quantum shift, we must...

*Be open to understanding the lost knowledge of the power and purpose of food.*

**Food has a power and purpose beyond scientific understanding!**

Recognize that plant foods, particularly in their raw form, possess the power to elevate the electrical frequency of our physical bodies, transforming them into containers of light.

The time has come to shift beyond the old food science paradigm of counting fats, calories, carbohydrates, and proteins, and embrace a new paradigm centered on consuming foods that contain lots of LIGHT ENERGY.

As I often say...

*Let LIGHT be your medicine and your medicine be LIGHT!*

To shift from the old fallen state of consciousness into the new, every cell of our physical bodies must be infused with highly charged electrical frequencies in order to empower them to shift into the higher frequencies of the New Earth. While this quantum shift will vary from person to person, the first dietary step we must all take is to eliminate lower frequency foods such as meat, dairy, and processed foods loaded with toxic chemicals—foods we were never originally designed to eat. These are foods that deplete our body's cellular electrical potential, block the flow of light, enslave our souls to the density of our physical bodies, and perpetuate disease and death.

Unfortunately, most educational institutions today teach a limited, myopic viewpoint of food, based on a food science theory that proposes a daily diet measured by the amount of fats, calories, carbohydrates, and proteins we consume. However, from a broader, more anthroposophical perspective, a few food scientists are challenging this outdated viewpoint. They are discovering that plant foods, grown through the power of photosynthesis, are infused with a range of phytochemicals that might represent the new frontier in food science.

*Photosynthesis* is a process by which green plants use sunlight, water, and carbon dioxide to create oxygen and energy in the form of complex carbohydrates. (Contrary to some beliefs, carbohydrates are not bad for us!) In Greek, photo means "light," and synthesis means "to make." Essentially, green plants use the light energy from the sun to produce phytochemicals, also known as phytonutrients.

*Phytochemicals* are chemical compounds found in plants that protect them against environmental threats such as bacteria, viruses, and fungi. Research now indicates that when we consume an array of plant-based phytochemicals, they may also protect us from these opportunistic threats. The more we consume, the greater our protection. Plant-based foods, such as fruits, vegetables, whole grains, nuts, seeds, and legumes, are abundant in phytochemicals, which also give them their color, flavor, and aroma.

While scientists have identified thousands of different phytochemicals, they are only beginning to understand the powerful roles these substances play in our overall health and wellbeing.

Debbie Krivitsky, director of clinical nutrition at the Cardiovascular Disease Prevention Center at Harvard-affiliated Massachusetts General Hospital, reports...

> "We're still just learning about phytochemicals. The science is ongoing. But they may help fight cancer and heart disease."

The American Institute for Cancer Research now recommends that everyone consider shifting to a mostly plant-based diet, as there is mounting evidence suggesting that phytochemicals, imbued with their rainbow of colors, may have the potential to...

- Aid the function of the immune system
- Protect cells and DNA from damage that may lead to cancer
- Slow the growth rate of some cancer cells
- Reduce inflammation
- Help regulate hormones

Andrea Murray, a food science specialist at the MD Anderson Research Division, states...

> "A plant-based diet strengthens your immune system to protect you against germs and microorganisms. ... Plants give your body what it needs to help fight off infection."

A healthy immune system is essential for reducing the risk of cancer, as well as most other diseases, because it can recognize and attack mutations in cells before they progress to disease.

Plant foods also reduce inflammation. The essential nutrients in plants work to resolve inflammation in your body. The same tiny phytochemicals and antioxidants that boost your immune system also circulate through your body, neutralizing toxins from pollution, processed food, bacteria, viruses, and more.

Andrea Murray also stated...

> "Antioxidants in plants grab all these so-called free radicals that can throw your body off balance. To reduce inflammation, it's important to eat plant-based and to listen to your body's signals for how foods work for you."

Prolonged inflammation can damage your body's cells and tissues and has been linked to cancer and other inflammatory diseases like arthritis. A plant-based diet may protect you because it removes some of the triggers of these diseases.

Stanford Medicine studies show that...

"Eating large amounts of brightly colored fruits and vegetables (yellow, orange, red, green, white, blue, purple), whole grains/cereals, and beans containing phytochemicals may decrease the risk of developing certain cancers as well as diabetes, hypertension, and heart disease. The action of phytochemicals varies by color and type of the food. They may act as antioxidants, nutrient protectors, or even prevent carcinogens (cancer-causing agents) from forming."

## Sources of Phytochemicals

Here's a partial list of phytochemicals found in foods:

- Allicin: Found in onions and garlic. Allicin blocks or eliminates certain toxins from bacteria and viruses.
- Anthocyanins: Found in red and blue fruits (such as raspberries and blueberries) and vegetables. They help slow the aging process, protect against heart disease and tumors, prevent blood clots, and fight inflammation and allergies.
- Bioflavonoids: Found in citrus fruits.
- Carotenoids: Found in dark yellow, orange, and deep green fruits and vegetables such as tomatoes, parsley, oranges, pink grapefruit, and spinach.
- Polyphenols (flavonoids, lignans, etc.): Found in fruits, vegetables, wine, olive oil, green tea, onions, apples, kale, and beans.
- Indoles: Found in broccoli, bok choy, cabbage, kale, Brussels sprouts, and turnips (also known as "cruciferous" vegetables). They contain sulfur and activate agents that destroy cancer-causing chemicals.

- Isoflavones: Found in soybeans and soybean products.
- Lignans: Found in flaxseed and whole grain products.
- Lutein: Found in leafy green vegetables. It may prevent macular degeneration and cataracts as well as reduce the risk of heart disease and breast cancer.
- Lycopene: Found primarily in tomato products. When cooked, it appears to reduce the risk of cancer and heart attacks.
- Phenolics: Found in citrus fruits, fruit juices, cereals, legumes, and oilseeds. It is thought to be extremely powerful and is studied for a variety of health benefits, including slowing the aging process, protecting against heart disease and tumors, and fighting inflammation, allergies, and blood clots.

## Foods Highest in Phytochemicals

Phytochemicals cannot be found in supplements and are only present in food. Foods high in phytochemicals include:

| | | |
|---|---|---|
| Broccoli | Olives | Soybeans |
| Berries | Tomatoes | Green tea |
| Soy nuts | Lentils | Apples |
| Pears | Cantaloupe | Cabbage |
| Turnips | Garlic | Brussels sprouts |
| Celery | Apricots | Bok choy |
| Carrots | Onions | Kale |
| Spinach | Seeds | Red wine |

## Foods Lowest in Phytochemicals

- Grains
- Legumes
- Nuts
- Seeds

While there are no recommended dietary allowances for the amount of phytochemicals, eating a variety of fruits and vegetables every day will guarantee you are getting adequate amounts.

We've been taught that our physical bodies are composed of approximately 100 trillion cells, and these cells are made up of about 100 trillion atoms, with atoms being 99.9999999 percent empty space. Some scientists believe that within this seemingly empty space is, in fact, LIGHT ENERGY! So, if this is true, and I believe it is, how is everything being held together within what appears to be the physical universe?

Most scientists believe that gravity holds everything in the physical universe together. However, new science postulates that everything is held together by an invisible electrical field of energy, not gravity! This new science is called *The Electric Universe Theory*.

**Our Physical Bodies Are LIGHT ENERGY**

The Electric Universe theorizes that the universe's true attractive force comes from invisible electric currents that not only surround our planet, our solar system, and our entire galaxy but also everything that appears to be matter. This theory suggests that what permeates space is a vast sea of ionized particles that create an enormous field of plasma. Plasma is known as the Fourth State of Matter; the others being solid, liquid, and gas.

Not only is our sun made up mostly of plasma, but plasma makes up over 99.9 percent of the visible universe. This network of plasma is so massive that it connects every galaxy in the universe in one single electrical circuit. This circuit not only conducts electricity over vast distances but transmits it faster than the speed of light!

If the Electric Universe Theory is true, and I believe it is, it will change everything we know about physics and reframe our understanding of the Cosmos and what we call matter.

Albert Einstein said...

> "Concerning matter, we have been all wrong. What we have called matter is energy whose vibration has been so lowered as to be perceptible to the senses. There is no matter."

Within this context, doesn't it make sense that a diet high in electrically charged Light Energy foods could be the secret to not only creating a healthy, sustainable life but also the secret to living a long life?

## Raw Fruits and Vegetables are Electrical by Nature

The trillions of cells that make up our organs, glands, and tissues are constantly conducting electrical currents to produce electricity for almost every function of the human body. Most scientists agree that our bodies, even when resting, can produce around 100 watts of power on average—enough electricity to power a light bulb!

Michael Hickner, an associate professor of materials science and engineering at Penn State, told Live Science,

> "Fruits and vegetables conduct electricity in the same way a salt solution will complete an electrical circuit."

To explore this theory further, I purchased something called a fruit clock—a device that doesn't require a traditional battery to run a clock.

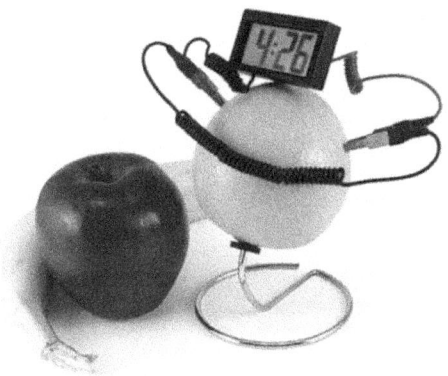

By placing two alternating (positive and negative) probes into most any type of raw fruit, it will literally run a clock simply because fruits and vegetables are high in electrolytes, especially organic sodium (salt)! But what happens if you place those same probes into a piece of cooked fruit? The clock won't run! That's because you've destroyed the enzyme-mineral component that helps to create electricity—organic sodium—a saline solution better known as salt!

It is also interesting to note that when fruits and vegetables are cooked, their phytochemical-nutrient-rich power becomes greatly diminished, as does the effect of antioxidants.

Dr. Robert Morse, author of The Detox Miracle Sourcebook, said...

> "When you eat foods picked fresh from nature, and eat them without cooking or processing them, the high electromagnetic energy of that food is transferred to your body and its cells."

The fact is: the trillions of cells that make up our organs, glands, and tissues are ELECTRICAL! What makes them electrical are the hundreds to thousands of mitochondria within our cells.

According to UCLA researchers, mitochondria are made up of many individual bioelectric units that generate energy like a Tesla electric car battery. Their main function is to generate the energy necessary to power our cells.

Essentially, they work like tiny little batteries and are responsible for keeping your "engine" running smoothly and efficiently. But there is more to mitochondria than energy production. Present in nearly all types of human cells, mitochondria are vital to our survival. They generate most of our adenosine triphosphate (ATP)—the energy currency of cells. Destroy the efficacy of mitochondria and you destroy life itself!

Science now knows that...

- When mitochondria are damaged, cells don't have enough energy to properly function and maintain themselves.
- Exposure to toxic substances such as prescription medications, vaccinations, wrong dietary choices, and environmental pollutants, coupled with living a sedentary lifestyle, creates mitochondrial dysfunction.
- Mitochondria become damaged by various mechanisms during our lifetime, mostly by free radicals and epigenetic changes.
- Various factors that damage mitochondria include nutrient deficiencies, toxic metals, environmental pollutants, most prescription drugs, and the overconsumption of alcohol.

- Damaged mitochondria send signals to cells, further disrupting proper cellular functioning. This leads to aging and eventually, a slow, painful death.

So, if you're ready to say YES to the *New Earth Diet*, you must first let go of the old paradigm of counting fats, calories, carbohydrates, and proteins in your daily diet and shift your focus to how much LIGHT ENERGY you are consuming every day.

Raw, electrically charged plant foods, filled with phytochemical/nutrients—foods that power up our cellular mitochondria—will not only enlighten you physically but also mentally, emotionally, and spiritually, simply because they are produced through the power of photosynthesis… the "light of the sun."

Then God said…

> "I give you every seed-bearing plant on the face of the whole earth and every tree that has fruit with seed in it. They will be yours for food."
> -Genesis 1:29

## THE THREE FUEL FOOD PLANS

Instead of following "man's" scientific way of eating that's based on fats, calories, carbohydrates, and protein, the recipes in this book are designed according to "nature's" way of eating, which is centered on the type of foods that will FUEL your cells with ENERGY, as detailed in my *New Earth Diet* book.

To begin your chosen Fuel Food Plan, remember... just as the grade of gasoline you burn in your car's engine affects our planet's environment in a positive or negative way, the grade of fuel you burn in your body's engine affects your body's environment in the same manner. Just as gasoline is classified by three grades: regular, midgrade, and premium, the foods you burn for fuel in your body's "engine" can also be classified by these same three grades.

The only question is—which one are you ready for?

The three classifications of fuel foods are...

**Regular Fuel (low octane)**
*The Beginner Fuel Food Plan*

80% Fruits & Veggies
20% Grains, Beans, Nuts & Seeds
50% Raw & 50% Cooked

**Midgrade Fuel (medium octane)**
*The Intermediate Fuel Food Plan*

80% Fruits & Veggies
10% Grains, Beans, Nuts & Seeds
80% Raw & 20% Cooked

**Premium Fuel (high octane)**
*The Master Fuel Food Plan*

95% Fruits & Veggies
5% Nuts & Seeds
100% Raw

Taking a little time to incorporate dietary changes can be very beneficial. Over the years, I have found that a drastic lifestyle change is more permanent when practiced over time. Obviously, strict adherence to the parameters outlined in The Premium Fuel Foods Plan will provide the greatest benefits but know that you don't have to be 100 percent on to win!

So, take your time as you transition back into what I believe to be our original diet; that is, unless you have some sort of major illness. If that's you, you may want to consider "passing go" and jump right into The Premium Fuel Foods Plan. With all of that said, let's get started!

## The Regular Fuel Foods Plan

- 80% Fruits and Veggies
- 20% Grains, Beans, Nuts, Seeds
- 50% Raw and 50% Cooked

This low octane fuel foods plan is for beginners. It is a transitional diet for those who have been eating an animal and/or processed-food diet. This plan is an all plant-based, organic, whole-foods diet that places emphasis on fruits and vegetables, gluten-free grains, beans, nuts, and seeds. It is animal-free, gluten-free, and processed-food free.

On this plan, you will follow the 80/20 Rule—80 percent fruits and vegetables, 20 percent grains and beans, and only a small portion of nuts and seeds. 50 percent of your food intake will be raw (uncooked), and 50 percent will be cooked.

In summary:
- No highly processed foods (with a few exceptions such as organic olive oil and apple cider vinegar).
- No animal meats, eggs, or dairy products.
- Eat all the organic fruits and vegetables you desire.
- Include a small portion of gluten-free grains, beans, nuts, and seeds.

You can include a small amount of Celtic Sea salt, organic olive oil, and natural sweeteners such as organic raw agave nectar, raw coconut nectar, or stevia.

**Eat seasonally.** Enjoy a mostly raw food diet in the spring and summer as they are the two warmest times of the year; eating lots of seasonal fruits, greens, and vegetables along with a very small portion of grains, beans, nuts, and seeds. Autumn and winter are the two coldest times of the year, so eating a more warming diet of cooked foods (unless you live in the tropics!), adding in steamed, roasted, or grilled vegetables, and a small portion of gluten-free grains, beans, nuts, and seeds, will serve you well.

**Follow nature's circadian rhythm.** From 4 a.m. until 12 noon, your body is in the elimination cycle. Fruits are cleansers so feel free to eat as much fruit as you want during this time or eat nothing at all until noon! From 12 noon until 8 p.m., your body is in the consumption cycle so feel free to eat as much Regular Fuel Foods as you want during this time. From 8 p.m. until 4 a.m., your body is in the assimilation cycle, at which time you will be consuming zero calories so your body has the time to assimilate what you've eaten.

**Follow food combining principles.** (1) Eat fruit only on an empty stomach, especially melons. (2) Never combine fruit with fat. (3) On occasion, you can combine fruit with leafy greens. (4) Avoid combining starches and proteins.

**Consume organic foods only.** Always choosing to only eat organic goes beyond simply supporting a more natural or eco-friendly approach to farming—it's about choosing foods that sustain both our health and the planet's. The contrast between organic and conventionally grown produce is stark, especially when considering the health implications, environmental impact, and long-term sustainability.

**Consume the right type of salt, oil, & sugar.** The importance of choosing the right types of salt, oil, and sugar for optimal health cannot be overstated. When you eat the wrong type of salt, oil, and sugar, your body will eventually send you an SOS (salt-oil-sugar) signal to warn you of a potential ecological threat! When choosing salt, always choose unrefined whole food salt such as Celtic Sea Salt. When choosing oil, always choose organic cold pressed olive oil high in polyphenols. When choosing sugar, always choose a whole food plant-based sugar such as organic raw agave or coconut sugar.

**Eat locally grown, seasonal produce**. Spending your money at a local farmer's market not only supports your health and the environment, but it also supports the livelihood of farmers in your community as well as the local economy. Eating during each season, spring, summer, autumn, and winter is a sustainable way of eating that has numerous health advantages.

# Regular Fuel Foods Menu Ideas

## What's for Breakfast?
100% Raw Fruits

The first meal of the day is "no food at all" or a fruitarian fare. Fruits are nature's cleansers, and from 4 a.m. until 12 noon, your body is in the elimination cycle. During this time, you would enjoy a bowl of seasonal fruit, a smoothie, or freshly prepared juice. Feel free to eat as much fruit as you want, or again, no food or calories at all until noon.

- ✓ Blend up a fruit smoothie with two cups of raw coconut water and any fruit in season. One of my favorites is very simple: fresh pineapple and raw coconut water. Add some greens or mint if you'd like.
- ✓ How about a delicious fruit salad with your favorite fruits in season? Enjoy it plain or drizzle with date sauce (four medjool dates, one cup water, and blend until creamy).
- ✓ Try blending one banana and several pitted dates with a cup of water; if it is wintertime and you want to warm yourself up, try adding a few shakes of cayenne pepper.
- ✓ Have a Green Smoothie. Blend a handful of stemmed kale or spinach with your choice of fresh organic, soluble-fiber fruit, such as mango, banana, or pear, and water. The soluble fiber makes for a creamy textured smoothie.
- ✓ Or, if you're like most and don't have a lot of time in the morning, simply add one to two tablespoons of your favorite green powder to your smoothie recipe of choice!
- ✓ Why not begin your day with one of my favorite juices? Juice three apples, one unpeeled lemon, a one-inch piece of fresh ginger, and

three beets. Then, if you want to take it up a "hot notch," add one-half habanero pepper. Great for flushing out your liver!
- ✓ Sometimes, I just like to keep it simple: one fruit at a time. Try a bowl of mangoes or papayas, grapes, peaches, pears, or some watermelon, whichever fruit is in season.

## What's for Lunch and Dinner?
50% Raw and 50% Cooked

- ✓ One of my favorite regular fuel foods meals is a small amount of gluten-free brown rice pasta tossed with crushed garlic, and salt. Add some freshly chopped basil and lots of cherry tomatoes cut in quarters. Toss again and then serve over a large bed of baby arugula.
- ✓ For a delicious Italian taste-bud delight, create a bountiful bowl of organic Roma tomatoes cut in quarters, tossed with Cannellini beans, salt, roasted red peppers, and garlic; all stacked high on a plate of chopped radicchio and Frise leaves.
- ✓ For a Greek delight, create a bowl of fava beans, thinly sliced red onion, cucumber, Roma tomatoes, pitted kalamata olives, several handfuls of romaine lettuce, and salt.
- ✓ Or, how about a Greek salad with sliced cucumbers, green bell peppers, tomatoes, red onion slivers, a dash of dill, and oregano, with a large serving of roasted veggies?
- ✓ If it's wintertime, enjoy a bowl of black beans, dash of cayenne pepper and cumin, tossed with escarole greens and lots of chopped avocado.
- ✓ How about a large bowl full of heirloom black rice, grilled or steamed asparagus, over a bed of finely chopped radicchio, tossed in your favorite dressing?

- ✓ How about a large arugula salad tossed with slices of sun-dried tomatoes, chopped olives, organic capers, tossed with olive oil and apple cider dressing, along with a bowl of your favorite plant-based cooked soup?
- ✓ For an Italian feast, try an Italian Potato Salad featuring fingerling potatoes, sliced red bell peppers, tossed in pressed garlic, and salt, then roasted in the oven until potatoes are slightly brown; then tossed with arugula. Delicious!
- ✓ For a Mexican feast, enjoy a large Salsa Wrap (salsa wrapped in a large lettuce leaf) with a bowl of Black Bean Soup. You can also use a tortilla made with brown rice.
- ✓ If it's cold outside and you want something to warm your bones, how about a bowl of Vegetable Bean Chili with your favorite salad?
- ✓ If it's springtime, enjoy a large salad with a bowl of your favorite asparagus soup.

## The Midgrade Fuel Foods Plan

- 90% Fruits and Vegetables
- 10% Grains, Beans, Nuts, Seeds
- 80% Raw and 20% Cooked

This medium octane fuel foods plan is a huge step-up from regular fuel foods. It's a diet for those who have been consuming regular fuel foods for several months and are ready to take a giant step up. Or it's for those who want to just go for it and skip the regular fuel foods plan entirely.

This plan consists of an all plant-based, whole-foods diet that places emphasis on equal proportions of fruits and vegetables, and a limited portion of gluten-free grains, beans, nuts, and seeds. It is animal-free, gluten-free, and processed-food free. On this plan, you will follow the 90/20 Rule—90 percent fruits and vegetables, 10 percent gluten-free grains, beans, and a small portion of nuts and seeds. 80 percent of your food intake will be raw (uncooked), and 20 percent will be cooked.

In summary:
- No highly processed foods (with a few exceptions such as organic olive oil and apple cider vinegar).
- No animal meats, eggs, or dairy products.
- Eat 90 percent organic fruits and vegetables (80% raw and 20% cooked).
- Include 10% gluten-free grains, beans, nuts, and seeds.
- Include a small amount of Celtic Sea salt, organic olive oil, and natural sweeteners such as organic raw agave nectar, raw coconut nectar, or stevia.
- Eat locally and seasonally (as previously outlined).
- Follow nature's circadian rhythm (as previously outlined).
- Follow food combining principles (as previously outlined).
- Eat organic produce only (as previously outlined).

# Midgrade Fuel Foods Menu Ideas

**What's for Breakfast?**
100% Fruit

For a fruitarian fare, start your day with your favorite seasonal fruits (or no calories at all until noon). Go ahead! Eat them, blend them, or juice them. You can use the same breakfast ideas from the Regular Fuel Foods Menu for your Midgrade Fuel Foods breakfast menu ideas.

Need a few more ideas? Try these!

- ✓ Try one of my Superfood Fruit Smoothies or use your own creative imagination. How about creating your smoothie with two to three different fruits such as a whole apple, banana, and orange along with two to three cups of water. Go ahead; blend the whole fruit, skin, seeds and all; the skins and seeds are loaded with phytonutrients. Add your favorite superfood raw, dehydrated juice powders such as Acai or goji berries, or raw green powder blend. Or simply add a handful of spinach!
- ✓ I love berries, and they are loaded with antioxidants, so how about a Berry Good Blend? Blend 1/2 cup of fresh organic raspberries, blueberries, strawberries, and blackberries with two to three cups of purified or coconut water; add a frozen banana and a superfood powder or juice blend. Go ahead; get creative!
- ✓ Take yourself to the tropics one morning with a Tropical Treat—blend one cup of fresh organic pineapple, mango, and papaya with lots of fresh young coconut water and coconut meat. Add a banana and blend!

- ✓ Have a Lean-Green Smoothie—for a highly concentrated dose of chlorophyll, blend a handful of stemmed dinosaur kale, one to two tablespoons of SevenPoint2 Greens with your choice of soluble-fiber fruit, such as mango or banana, and three cups purified water or raw coconut water.

## What's for Lunch and Dinner?
80% Raw and 20% Cooked

- ✓ How about a large bowl of your favorite leafy greens, topped with a small portion of steamed or roasted fingerling potatoes, tossed with pressed garlic and a dash of rosemary powder?
- ✓ For a simple yet delicious meal in a bowl, create a bountiful bowl of your favorite chopped raw veggies, a few steamed or roasted fingerling potatoes, tossed with a dash of rosemary powder, chopped parsley, mint, dill, green onions, avocado, and tomatoes.
- ✓ Try a large bowl of leafy greens topped with your favorite steamed veggies and a drizzle of your favorite salad dressing?
- ✓ For a delicious Italian delight, create a bountiful bowl of Roma tomatoes cut in quarters, tossed with roasted red peppers, chopped basil, garlic, stacked high on a plate of chopped radicchio and Frise leaves—drizzled with your favorite salad dressing, or simply use a dash of balsamic vinegar.
- ✓ If it's springtime, you might enjoy a large asparagus salad featuring lots of steamed or raw asparagus pieces, sliced cherry tomatoes, diced Valencia oranges, chopped shallots, all tossed in your favorite salad dressing, or simply tossed in lemon juice and tarragon.
- ✓ Enjoy a large watercress salad tossed with a ripe papaya, along with a bowl of your favorite soup. Or, simply enjoy a bowl of "energy

soup" made with a handful of baby greens, one to two cups of sunflower sprouts, half an avocado, one whole apple (peel, seeds and all), and raw coconut water.

- ✓ For an autumn feast, how about a small baked yam drizzled in organic raw agave nectar, with a large raw veggie chop salad on the side?
- ✓ Or, how about a raw Greek salad with sliced cucumbers, green bell peppers, Roma tomatoes, red onion slivers, a dash of dill and oregano, along with a side of steamed veggies?
- ✓ If it's wintertime, enjoy a large, chopped veggie salad with a hot bowl of veggie soup.

## The Premium Fuel Foods Plan

- 95% Fruits and Vegetables
- 5% Nuts and Seeds
- 100% Raw

This diet is for those who are ready for mastership. This plan consists of a plant-based, organic, 100 percent raw food diet that places emphasis on fruits, dark leafy greens, non-starchy vegetables, and a very small portion of nuts and seeds. This diet is animal-free, dairy-free, grain-free, bean-free, and starch-free. Over time, this plan will clean the accumulated toxins and acids out of your body like no other food program out there.

This is because of the cleansing and regenerating power of electrically-powered fruit—the original food you were designed to eat. This plan is for those who are ready to move out of survival adaptation and go for the highest state of health and wellbeing possible—a return to Eden! Try it, even if it's just for 30 days, and see what I mean!

**On this plan, you will follow the 95/5 Plan**
That means, 95 percent fruits and vegetables, and 5 percent nuts and seeds—100 percent raw. The main difference between midgrade fuel and premium fuel is that you'll be increasing your intake of fruits and vegetables, eliminating all starchy foods such as potatoes, and eating everything in its raw, living state.

This means:

- No processed foods (with a few whole food exceptions).
- No animal meats, eggs, or dairy.
- No grains or beans.
- Eat 95 percent organic fruits and vegetables—100% raw.
- Include a small amount of Celtic Sea salt and organic olive oil.
- Eat locally and seasonally (as previously outlined).
- Follow nature's circadian rhythm (as previously outlined).
- Follow food combining principles (as previously outlined).
- Eat organic produce only (as previously outlined).

And no! You don't have to spend hours in the kitchen prepping, dehydrating, and preparing fancy raw-food meals; that is, unless you want to. All you do is pick, peel, and eat—just as if you were living out in nature.

Simply keep in mind that the reason you eat is to fuel the trillions of cells that swim throughout the waters of your body with foods that supply them with lots of energizing fuel. Again, fruits, greens, and vegetables, along with a small number of nuts and seeds, are the premium fuel foods! To show you how simple it is, here's a sample week of menu ideas.

## Premium Fuel Foods Menu Ideas

### What's for Breakfast?
100% Fruit

Seasonal fruits are the main fuel for breakfast. It's the time of the day your body needs to not only eliminate any toxic, accumulated waste, but it's also the time every cell in your body requires the extra high-octane energy that only fruits can give.

- ✓ Enjoy as much freshly prepared juice or smoothies as you want for breakfast.
- ✓ If it's summertime, eat as much watermelon as you want.
- ✓ Have my favorite Banana Date Smoothie: Blend two bananas with three medjool dates in sixteen ounces of water. Simply delicious.
- ✓ What about a Tropical Delight? Blend one large mango, one banana, and one small papaya with one to two cups of raw coconut water.
- ✓ How about a Berry Good Smoothie today? Blend one banana, one cup blueberries, one cup strawberries, one cup raspberries with the juice of three oranges.
- ✓ Try a Mango Mania Smoothie today: Blend three mangoes, one banana, with sixteen ounces of coconut water and enjoy.
- ✓ At least once a week, I enjoy a very simple Pineapple Coconut

Smoothie for breakfast: I simply blend 1-quart pineapple pieces with 20 ounces raw coconut water.

- ✓ How about a simple blend of freshly prepared orange juice with lots of strawberries? It's one of my favorites.

**What's for Lunch and Dinner?**
100% Raw

Whether you're eating out or in, leafy green salads and raw soups are the high-octane fuel fare for lunch and dinner. Use your imagination, choose your favorite veggies in season, and create your own. Or choose a premium fuel salad and/or raw soup from my New Earth Cookbook!

- ✓ Enjoy a Zucchini Linguini Salad! That's right, "raw zucchini pasta," and it's simple to make. Using a paring knife, shave long strips of organic raw zucchini, or simply use a Spirooli Spiral Slicer. Simply place your zucchini pasta in a bowl and toss it with pressed garlic, freshly chopped basil, and lots of cherry tomatoes sliced in half, all tossed with pesto, and served on a bed of arugula.

- ✓ If you're having lunch or dinner out, have a large Caesar salad (hold the anchovies!) featuring Romaine lettuce, tomatoes, and avocado tossed in a creamy raw cashew dressing. (1 cup raw cashews, juice of one large lemon, 2 cups water, 3 cloves garlic, salt, then blended in a high-power blender).

- ✓ How about being creative and making a bowl of raw soup in your blender and a bowl of salad as a meal from the ingredients that you love the most?

- ✓ If it's summertime, how about having a mono fruit meal for lunch? Eat as many bananas, or mangoes, or peaches as you want! Or, have an Acai Green or Green and Lean Smoothie found in my *New Earth Cookbook*.

- ✓ Enjoy a bowl of pineapple gazpacho raw soup (raw pineapple chunks, tomatoes, basil, jalapeno pepper, apple cider vinegar, salt, and blended) served with a small, chopped veggie salad, tossed with your favorite dressing.
- ✓ How about a Greek salad tonight (Romaine lettuce, tomatoes, green peppers, red onion, and salt) with a bowl of raw cucumber-dill soup (use your imagination and blender!)?
- ✓ If it's springtime, how about having a delicious salad bowl of your favorite greens tossed in your favorite dressing, served with a bowl of raw tomato basil soup (use your imagination and blender!)?
- ✓ Or, how about a salsa lettuce wrap (place your favorite salsa in a butternut lettuce leaf) with a bowl of raw gazpacho soup?

So go ahead, Enlighten Yourself! Eat your way to wellness! I did, and so can you!

## Drink Lots of Enlightenment Juices

One of the fastest ways to restore your internal environment to a perfect state of health and wellbeing is to juice your way to wellness! Drinking freshly extracted green juices every day is like having a blood transfusion from nature's hospital. In fact, this is what I did approximately 40 years ago to recover from my internal environmental crisis. After reading Dr. Norman Walker's book, Fresh Vegetable and Fruit Juices, I put my new juice machine to the test.

For 90 days, I drank two quarts of various vegetable and fruit juices along with eating lots of fruits during the day and a green leafy salad in the early evening. My family thought I had lost my mind, but what I had truly lost was an immune-deficient, disease-ridden body. The germ that had made my body its home had had its environment altered. With no more acidic food supply, it had no other choice but to pack up and go someplace else.

Fresh vegetable and fruit juices provide the body with an enormous amount of nutrients and phytonutrients for cleansing and rebuilding. It is the body's innate intelligence (sometimes referred to as the healer within) that knows how to restore ecological balance when given the proper nutrients. What I discovered is that if you provide your body with the right materials in the right amount, this intelligence knows exactly how to go about restoring your health.

Citrus fruits are generally peeled, and many of us pick away at the white tissue surrounding the juicy segments to clean it all away. Remember that both the skin and the white tissue are especially rich in flavonoids—a phytonutrient that has great nutritional value. The parts that we generally throw away have been found to be anticarcinogenic, anti-inflammatory, and have free-radical scavenging properties. While I don't include the peel in smoothies, I always include it when making juice.

So go ahead! Enlighten yourself! Juice your way to wellness! I did, and so can you!

## Drink Lots of Enlightenment Smoothies

Science has recently discovered that plants convert solar energy into complex chemical compounds called phytochemicals, also called phytonutrients, contained in plant foods such as fruits, berries, vegetables, nuts, and seeds. When you plant a seed into rich soil, it uses the power of the sun to draw nutrients from the soil to convert inorganic substances into organic substances. In turn, these nutrients power all living organisms on earth.

Currently, phytochemical-nutrients are being used interchangeably to describe the biologically active compounds of plants considered to have a highly beneficial effect on human health. These compounds, such as anthocyanins, which are flavonoid pigments that give every plant its color, have been found to exhibit diversified physiologic and pharmacologic effects.

In essence, fruits and vegetables have the power to color you healthy! Thus, to get a healthy variety of phytochemical-nutrients every day, think color! Fruit and vegetable pigments are compounds that give them their color. Different pigments have different functions and react in various ways. Blending fruits and vegetables of different colors every day gives your body a wide range of valuable nutrients (phytonutrients) that science now knows will protect you from almost every chronic disease known.

Consuming a vibrant rainbow of fruits and vegetables every day fuels your body with a wide range of valuable phytochemical-nutrients that science now knows will protect you from almost every chronic disease known. The peel contains more than four times as much fiber as the fruit inside, and more flavonoids with anticancer, anti-diabetic, and anti-inflammatory properties. A 2004 study on animals suggests that these nutrients may even reduce harmful LDL cholesterol better than some prescription drugs. The peels can be a little strong for a smoothie, so I personally grate and sprinkle the peels, called zest, stir it in or top it off!

Thus, one of the best ways to be assured of getting phytochemical-nutrients, such as flavonoids, bioflavonoids, or carotenoids, is to simply blend and drink it all—seeds, skin, and flesh. These nutritional powerhouses exhibit a cornucopia of health-giving benefits.

> **Red Fruits and Vegetables** are known for lycopene, quercetin, and other antioxidants that neutralize free radicals, regulate blood pressure, and reduce the risk of prostate cancer, among other things. Nature's red fruits include strawberries, cranberries, and watermelon. Red vegetables include red peppers, radishes, and beets.
>
> **Orange and Yellow Fruits and Vegetables** contain beta-carotene, zeaxanthin, potassium, and vitamin C. They are abundant in antioxidants and other phytonutrients that are good for your skin, joints, eyes, and heart and also decrease your risk of cancer. Nature's orange and yellow fruits include oranges, mangoes, and peaches. Orange and yellow vegetables include sweet potatoes, corn, and pumpkin.
>
> **Blue and Purple Fruits and Vegetables** contain lutein, resveratrol, and various flavonoids. Evidence indicates that these purple pigments protect our brains as we age, strengthen our immune system, support healthy digestion, and have anti-carcinogenic properties. Blue and purple fruits include blueberries, plums, and grapes. Blue and purple vegetables include eggplant, cabbage, and endive.
>
> **White Fruits and Vegetables** contain allicin, an antifungal compound found in the garlic and onion family, and beta-

glucans and lignans, which have powerful immune-boosting properties. These powerful phytochemical-nutrients are also known to balance hormones and reduce the risk of colon, breast, prostate, and hormone-related cancers. Nature's white fruits include bananas, pears, and dates. White vegetables include onions, potatoes, and cauliflower.

**Green Fruits and Vegetables** contain ample stores of chlorophyll, lutein, folate, and calcium. They neutralize free radicals, strengthen the immune system, regulate blood pressure, and reduce cancer risks. Does it sound familiar yet? Green fruits include avocados, kiwi, and honeydew melons. Green vegetables include leafy greens, asparagus, and peas.

Just remember that the "whole" food is greater than the sum of the parts. Listing the scientific properties of the known nutrients cannot give you the whole story of the plant itself. The "disease-fighting" properties of phytonutrients are, indeed, just the tip of a highly charged, transformational iceberg.

So go ahead! Enlighten yourself! Blend your way to wellness! I did, and so can you!

# AIR
## Breathe To Enlighten Yourself

You can go for weeks without food, days without water, but only a few minutes without breathing. Breathing has such an immediate impact on your mind and body that even the act of inhaling versus exhaling affects your nervous system differently.

Day-in and day-out, we are all breathing, without thinking and for most of us, without any effort. So why should we care about our breath? Most of us have been taught that the purpose of breathing is to draw oxygen into our lungs through the air we breathe in and to release carbon dioxide in the air we breathe out. Then, once it enters our lungs, the oxygen passes into our blood where it is carried by hemoglobin (a red protein responsible for transporting oxygen in the blood) to our cells, which uses it to generate energy.

Many of our health problems, which generally goes undiagnosed, can often be traced back to shallow breathing. But when we learn how to breathe correctly, our breath can have a powerful influence on our overall health.

You can often determine your dominant nervous system state simply by placing your finger underneath your nostrils and exhaling. Reduced rate breathing can stimulate a rest and digest, parasympathetic nervous system state to help with sleep, stress, and anxiety. Rapid, pulsed breathing stimulates a sympathetic nervous system response to increase energy, prepare for exercise, or boost the body's natural defenses.

Diaphragmatic breathing massages the vagus nerve and reduces heart rate, lowers blood pressure, and reduces stress. Severe respiratory conditions like asthma can be successfully managed by increasing $CO_2$ levels in the blood. Breathing can also help reduce the fear of public speaking, improve digestion, reduce insomnia, lower stress, anxiety, and overwhelm.

Like the wind circulates air throughout our planet's atmosphere, our breath circulates air throughout our body's atmosphere, cleansing, oxygenating, and bringing life to every cell of our physical bodies.

Sadly, most of us have forgotten the transformational power of our breath. We have become a nation of stress-driven, sedentary-shallow chest breathers. Most of us are taking a minimal amount of breath into our lungs, generally by drawing air into the chest area using the intercostals muscle instead of through the lungs via our diaphragm.

Most chest breathers breathe shallowly throughout the day and are almost always unaware of it. Shallow breathing causes a build-up of carbon dioxide in the blood, which causes the blood to become oxygen deprived.

When we take a full deep breath, our diaphragm (a dome-shaped structure that acts as a natural partition between our heart and lungs and organs) moves through its entire range downward to massage and oxygenate the liver, stomach, and other organs and tissues below it, and upward to massage and oxygenate the heart. Also, with a full deep breath, the diaphragm moves farther down into the abdomen, assisting our lungs to expand more completely into the chest cavity.

This means that with each breath, more oxygen is taken in, and more carbon dioxide is released. It also means that with each full, deep breath, we're increasing blood flow and peristalsis and pumping the lymph more efficiently throughout our lymphatic system.

The lymphatic system, which is an important part of our immune system, has no other means of pumping the lymph other than muscular movements, including the movements of breathing.

Consider that…

> *Science has proven that cancer is anaerobic, it does not survive in high levels of oxygen.*

Shortness of breath and heart disease are directly linked—the heart goes into spasm when it is deprived of oxygen.

Studies have shown that there is a high correlation between high blood pressure and poor breathing. Most emotional issues, including anxiety and depression, result from the nervous system being out of balance. Breathing drives the nervous system.

Optimal breathing helps to promote weight loss. Oxygen burns fat and calories. Breathing well is the key to sleeping well and waking up feeling rested. Breathing provides 99% of your energy. Without energy, nothing works.

Virtually every health condition and human activity is improved with optimal breathing.

Clinical studies prove that oxygen, wellness, and life-span are totally dependent on proper breathing. Lung volume is a primary marker for how long you will live.

Again, the most pervasive reason we have forgotten how to breath properly is that we have been strongly influenced and impacted by our sedentary modern-day society. We all need to move! Movement causes us to breathe, and our breath is the fuel that will create that healthier, happier, more alkaline you that you were designed to be.

> **Did you know…**
>
> **Breathing can change your blood pH (acid to alkaline) in minutes. No food, exercise or supplement acts as quickly.**

## Breathing Practices

Learning to develop the power of your breath is of the utmost importance. It is an indispensable aid to superior health, peak performance, and life extension.

Let's try a few.

### Breathe to Relax
Sit comfortably with eyes open or shut. With mouth closed, inhale and exhale several times. Next, begin slowly exhaling through your

nose, counting to seven, starting at the top of your chest, moving down through your mid-torso and into your diaphragm. Pause for seven counts. Begin inhaling slowly through your nose, counting to seven, starting at your diaphragm, expanding your belly, then your mid-torso, and lastly the top of your chest. Pause for seven counts and exhale as before. Repeat 5-10 times.

Once again, sit in a comfortable position. With mouth closed, breathe in and out through your nose as fast and equally as possible. Continue for 10-15 seconds at first, and then as you become more accustomed to this type of rapid breath, increase it to one full minute. This breath practice is a very ancient belly breath that energizes you while toning the abdomen and massaging the internal organs and lymph system. This type of breathing activates the lungs, neck, chest and abdomen.

**Breathe to Slim Down**
If you find it's tough to exercise on a regular basis, try deep breathing exercises, which can be done anytime, anywhere. Deep breathing greatly assists in facilitating weight loss due to the fact that large amounts of oxygen cause the chemical reactions in your body to take place much faster, thus you burn more calories than you take in.

This in turn speeds up your metabolism and makes you burn more body fat. Body fat is also eliminated with the release of carbon dioxide. In a relatively short time you'll not only feel the difference, you'll see the difference. The answer is to simply breathe deeply and do it often throughout the day.

Always remember, whenever you feel stressed, breathe! If stress isn't managed properly, your body will burn glycogen, not fat, for that extra energy needed. Just by triggering a relaxation response by using a few deep breaths, your body is encouraged to burn fat instead.

The following deep breathing exercises can be performed sitting down or standing up: Begin by blowing as much air as you can out of your lungs through your mouth. When you feel as though you don't have any more air to expel, give it one more thrust, completely emptying your lungs. Relax for a few seconds. Close your mouth and quickly inhale through your nose, pulling as much air into your lungs as possible, always focusing your breath onto the area of the diaphragm (the diaphragm is located just below the sternum in the "V" formed by the rib cage).

As the diaphragm expands, the lower abdomen should rise slightly, followed by the chest (note that if you're not making a noise, you're most likely not doing it right). Continue to steadily pull the air in as deeply as you can, completely filling your lungs.

When you feel as if you've taken in all the air you possibly can, open your mouth and take a final gasp of air in through your mouth. Hold for 7-10 seconds. Open your mouth wide and exhale from the diaphragm with a quick, explosive breath through your mouth. Again, you should breathe out hard enough that you are able to hear the noise as you force the air from deep inside.

Continue exhaling, completely emptying your lungs. As you blow the air out, roll your stomach in and up. This is the most important step, particularly if you want to flatten your stomach, tone your abdominal muscles and oxygenate every cell of your body.

My favorite deep-breathing exercise is rebounding on a mini-trampoline. And it's easy to fit it into your daily routine. I often rebound several times a day while listening to my favorite music. Some scientists have even concluded that jumping on a mini trampoline is one of the most effective exercises yet devised by man, especially because of the effect rebounding has on the lymph system.

Lymph fluid moves through channels called "vessels" that are filled with one-way valves, so the lymph always moves in the same direction. The main lymph vessels run up the legs, up the arms and up the torso. This is why the vertical up and down movement of rebounding is so effective to pump the lymph.

The mini trampoline subjects the body to gravitational pulls ranging from zero at the top of each bounce to 2 to 3 times the force of gravity at the bottom, depending on how high a person is rebounding. This gravitation pull has the power to pump the lymph like nothing else. Then, when you add deep-breathing exercises to your rebounding bounce, the alkalizing effect goes off the chart!

Just be sure to consume lots of organic fruit, green leafy vegetables, and sprouts. This is because your body needs adequate amounts of high-quality glucose to maintain high oxygen levels as the whole purpose of oxygen is to combine with glucose to manufacture ATP (adenosine triphosphate) in the cells, which powers the whole process of life. Most people who tend to be shallow breathers are low in high-quality glucose because the extra oxygen simply cannot be used.

This is why the *New Earth Diet* consists of 80 percent fruits and green-leafy vegetables.

## Breathe the Breath of God

The most profound thing to understand about the power of your breath is to understand that your breath is the breath of God who is breathing you!

The book of Genesis tells us that, in the beginning, "a mighty wind" swept over the darkness of the abyss (1:2). And out of the chaos, this mighty wind, which was literally the breath of God, breathed everything into existence… Including YOU!

> "Then the Lord God formed man out of the dust of the ground and breathed into his nostrils the breath of life; and man became a living soul."
>
> -Genesis 2:7

In essence, God never left us. But because we live in a sensory physical universe, our senses have dulled our conscious connection with God, which is what causes most of earthly problems.

But if we would wake up from our mortal slumber, we will come to realize that…

> *We are not separate from our Creator, or anyone, or anything that only appears to be outside of us. It's merely an illusion.*

Albert Einstein said…

> "Concerning matter, we have been all wrong. What we have called matter is energy, whose vibration has been so lowered as to be perceptible to the senses. There is no matter."

He also said…

> "What we call reality is an illusion, albeit a very persistent one."

So, if this is true, and I believe it is, is it possible that God's breath has the power to breathe every sickness and disease out of our bodies? I believe, YES… because it happened to me!

As detailed in Chapter One, I was sick and almost died from an unknown viral/bacterial infection. Despite seven days of the strongest intravenous antibiotics possible, my white-blood-cell count kept dropping. My physicians had no clue to the cause and, therefore, no cure for my problem. I had been given 24 hours to live if my white-blood-cell didn't start going up.

Later that night, alone in my isolation room, my life would change forever. As the stillness of the night wrapped itself around me, I became consciously aware of the subtle breeze of my breath as it moved in and out of my nostrils.

Then suddenly, out of the darkness, an angelic presence appeared out of a golden halo of light above me. It was beyond anything I had ever seen before. We began having an intimate, yet silent communication.

> With fixed eyes, I cried out, "I'm dying, and they have no cure for me!"

> The angelic presence replied, "How can they possibly have a cure when they don't understand your real problem?"

"So, what's my real problem?" I asked.

"The illusion that you're separate from God, from nature, and from everything and everyone around you. If you will stay focused upon your breath, the breath of God who breathed you into physical existence, you will live!"

And so, I did. For hours!

The next morning, I woke up out of a deep sleep with a visceral knowing that it truly is the breath of God who is breathing me. God wasn't in a far-off place called Heaven judging my every move, as I had been taught in church. God was a subtle, yet dynamic power and presence within me, breathing me, into me!

A few hours after the lab technician had taken more blood, my physician walked into my room with my family with a huge smile. He said...

"I have no idea what happened in the night, but it's a miracle! Your white-blood-cell count is normal!"

A few weeks later, I began calling this way of breathing, "The Breath of Translation." To translate means to change to a different substance, form, or appearance. And that, I did! But only after I viscerally realized that...

"God is the very breath I breathe!" GOD IS!

So go ahead! Enlighten yourself! Breathe your way to wellness! I did, and so can you!

# FIRE
## Sunbathe to Enlighten Yourself

The energy of the sun is related to the fire element. The sun is a huge ball of fire that fuels every aspect of life on our planet. Fundamentally, fire is fuel. It's solar-powered energy creates electricity, petrol, wood, coal, or whatever else, but essentially, it is fire that fuels everything, including your body. This is because, like plants, mitochondria (the powerhouse within our cells) have the ability to photosynthesize, or to convert light into energy. Thus, sunlight exposure increases ATP levels and cellular respiration, giving our cells more energy.

Today, however, most of us have lost our personal relationship with the sun and its relationship with us. Throughout the history of time, we've gone from worshipping it to shunning it, both in the religious sense as well as in the bronzed sense. While every living thing upon our planet is dependent upon the light of the sun, we've been made to believe that it's our enemy.

Some believe that the sun is something to be shunned and avoided and that sunbathing, and an ancient practice known as sun-gazing are dangerous practices that can destroy our retinas, age our skin, and often cause skin cancer. Current scientific research, however, exposes these narrow archaic myths.

Let us now reconsider ending our on-again, off-again relationship with sunlight and open ourselves to an understanding of its importance towards achieving a state of health and enlighten state of wellbeing.

# EAT LIGHT

National Library of Medicine reports studies proving that sun exposure has positive effects on immune function and cardio-metabolic health, working through both vitamin D and non-vitamin D pathways. Any positive non-vitamin D pathway effects of sun exposure will not be apparent in vitamin D supplementation trials and may explain the discrepancies between observational studies and clinical trials. In essence, our bodies must have natural sunlight exposure.

Michael Holick, M.D., the world's foremost authority on vitamin D and the healing power of natural sunlight, says that adequate amounts of sensible sun exposure during childhood not only maximizes the bone health of children but may even decrease their risk of many chronic diseases in later life including type-1 diabetes, multiple sclerosis, rheumatoid arthritis, and common cancers.

In his book, The UV Advantage, Dr. Holick states how vitamin D deficiencies can cause prostate cancer, breast cancer, cervical cancer, osteoporosis, rickets, and various other diseases. According to two recent studies, he recommends that increasing vitamin D intake through natural sunlight and diet may decrease a person's risk of contracting breast cancer by 50 percent and of contracting colorectal cancer by more than 65 percent.

Several studies have shown that exposure to natural sunlight increases the number of white blood cells in the body, which plays the leading role in defending against invasions of bacteria and foreign organisms. Because of the increase in white blood cell activity after sunlight exposure, a person's ability to fight infections is greatly increased along with the body's ability to stop the reproduction of viruses.

This is astounding!

While it's important that we absorb the rays of the sun every day, like most anything else, sunbathing can be overdone. The sun must be treated with great respect. The skin must be properly conditioned to sunlight. Too much sun during the wrong time of day is unwise. The best time to absorb the rays of the sun is before 10am or after 3pm—a time when the UV rays are less potent. Start with 15 minutes either early morning (9am) or late afternoon (4pm). Add 15 more minutes each day until you have a healthy, bronze tan. Remember, the less clothing or covering the better. So, when it comes to properly absorbing sunlight, remember to always EAT LIGHT!

Microbiome is the collection of all microorganisms, bacteria, fungi, and viruses. Well, we used to think about the bacteria that colonized humans as bad. We always thought of them as pathogens, and we wanted to try to destroy them and thought that was the real benefit of antibiotics. But now science recognizes that there also are good microbes, or commensal microbes, that provide needed help to the human and similarly would provide benefit to the environmental source.

So for humans, bacteria that live in your gut help in the digestion of food, and bacteria that live on your skin help to break down the lipids to produce natural moisturizing factor for your skin. These microbes that live on your skin or in your gut also are wonderful in providing colonization resistance. They're basically taking up all the space so that the pathogens that might want to try to invade humans don't have the opportunity, and that's really our greatest protection against microbes that want to colonize us but don't help in our health.

A new paper underscores that the importance of creating and maintaining healthy bacteria in the mouth is an essential step in understanding how oral health affects systemic disease. These data suggest that management of the tongue microbiome by regular cleaning together with adequate dietary intake of nitrate provide an opportunity for the improvement of resting blood pressure. The paper appears today in Frontiers in Cellular and Infection Microbiology.

Nathan, Bryan, Ph.D., said...

> "Nitric oxide is one of the most important signaling molecules produced in the human body."

As N.O. is a ubiquitous signaling molecule, the systemic effects of orally produced bacteria may have other significant effects on human health beyond maintenance of blood pressure. We know one cannot be well without an adequate amount of N.O. circulating throughout the body. Yet, the very first thing over 200 million Americans do each day is use an antiseptic mouthwash, which destroys the 'good bacteria' that helps to create the N.O. These once thought good habits may be doing more harm than good. Another oral microbiome destroying factor is fluoride found in our drinking water and various toothpastes!

The demonstration that the presence of N.O. producing bacteria in the oral cavity can help maintain normal blood pressure gives us another target to help the more than 100 million Americans living with high blood pressure. Manipulation of the human microbiome as a therapeutic target for disease management is on the near horizon. Screening the oral microbiome of resistant hypertensive patients may provide new insights into the etiology of their hypertension. Two out of three patients prescribed high blood pressure medication do not have their blood pressure adequately managed. This may provide an explanation as to why. None of the currently FDA-approved drugs for management of hypertension are targeted towards these N.O. producing bacteria.

There is enormous interest and research in the microbiome but most of the focus is on the gut microbiome. It is time we focus on the most proximal part of our gastrointestinal system, the mouth. The oral cavity is an attractive target for probiotic and/or prebiotic therapy because of the ease of access. The potential to restore the oral flora to provide N.O. production is a completely new paradigm for N.O. biochemistry and physiology as well as to cardiovascular medicine and dentistry.

These studies provide new insights into the host-oral microbiome symbiotic relationship. If we are going to make a leap forward in health, we need to take another look at boosting oral health as it relates to N.O. production and the role it plays in disease or find safe and effective therapeutic strategies to recapitulate N.O. production in the oral cavity," he said.

According to Dr. Nathan Bryan, the first step to rebuilding your oral microbiome is to stop using mouthwash, stop drinking fluoridated water, and stop using fluoride toothpaste!

Now, let's dive into the power of sunlight and healthy gut microbes! On the surface, sunlight and gut microbes may seem to have nothing in common… but think again!

A skin-gut axis has been discovered that links exposure to sunlight directly to changes in our gut microbiome which, according to the Frontiers in Microbiology study, could also lead to a more varied collection of gut bacteria.

The Canadian researchers have been studying the effects of UV light on the gut's microorganisms because they discovered that low levels of sun exposure, insufficient levels of vitamin D, and a lack of microbiome diversity, have all been linked to certain inflammatory health conditions, such as inflammatory diseases such as bowel disease and multiple sclerosis.

> "The results of this study have implications for people who are undergoing UVB phototherapy and identifies a novel skin-gut axis that may contribute to the protective role of UVB light exposure in inflammatory diseases like MS and IBD."
> –Prof. Bruce Vallance

Else Bosman, a researcher and doctoral candidate in the Department of Experimental Medicine at the University of British Columbia, said…

> "This is the first study to find a direct effect of UVB on intestinal microbes," said The findings also point to the important role that vitamin D, which is produced when UV rays hit the skin, appears to play in "maintaining healthy gut microbe composition"

To explore the impact of sunlight on the microbiome, the researchers recruited 21 healthy women whose average age was 28. At the start of the study, the volunteers had their vitamin D levels measured, and also had stool samples examined to determine the makeup of their microbiomes, the collection of microorganisms that populate the gut. The women were then exposed to a narrow band of UVB rays three times in one week. (UVA and UVB are the two main types of UV light that reach the Earth from the sun.) Because the study took place in winter in Canada, all of the women had little sun exposure otherwise. Some, however, had been taking supplements to keep their vitamin D levels up; most of the women who weren't supplementing had "insufficient" levels of vitamin D.

At the end of the week, the women had their vitamin D levels and stool samples checked again. Vitamin D levels increased in the majority of the volunteers. The women who had low levels of vitamin D at the beginning of the study now had normal levels and, intriguingly, their microbiomes had become more diverse.

**Sunlight Lowers Blood Pressure**
Research carried out at the Universities of Southampton and Edinburgh shows that sunlight alters levels of the small messenger molecule, nitric oxide (NO), in the skin and blood, reducing blood pressure.

Professor of Experimental Medicine and Integrative Biology at the University of Southampton, Martin Feelisch, comments...

> "N.O. along with its breakdown products, known to be abundant in skin, is involved in the regulation of blood pressure. When exposed to sunlight, small amounts of N.O. are transferred from

the skin to the circulation, lowering blood vessel tone; as blood pressure drops, so does the risk of heart attack and stroke."

The results suggest that UV exposure dilates blood vessels, significantly lowers blood pressure, and alters N.O. metabolite levels in the circulation, without changing vitamin D levels. Further experiments indicate that pre-formed stores of N.O. in the upper skin layers are involved in mediating these effects.

**Benefits of Sun-Gazing**
Sun-gazing is a term broadly applied to an ancient meditative practice of staring directly at the sun at sunrise and/or sunset. Some believe this practice is dangerous while others believe it's one of the highest spiritual practices we can do. This practice takes place during the first or last 30 minutes of the day so that UV radiation is at its minimum. If great caution is used, i.e. staring at the sun for shorter periods of time, such as five minutes, then gradually working up to longer amounts of time, retina damage to the eyes can be avoided. As an interesting sidebar, sun-gazing during a solar eclipse is not recommended.

While there has not been any scientific evidence to substantiate the beneficial claims of sun-gazing, there are reports that suggest gazing can provide the sun-gazer with a sense of physical, mental, emotional, and spiritual wellbeing. Some even report a decrease in irritability, anger, and frustration, and an increase in memory. Others even claim a complete relief from almost every disease known.

Sun-gazing is often practiced with bare feet in direct contact with the earth. You begin by staring directly at the rising sun for ten seconds then adding an additional ten seconds to the total sun-gazing time each consecutive day until you are staring at the sun for 45 minutes. In six months, some have experienced the feeling of hunger dissipate, and after ten months others claim that they never need to eat again!

In other words, they are eating light; sunlight has become the primary food they're burning for energy. It is alleged that after 45 minutes of sun-gazing, one would be full of light energy, just like a solar-charged battery, with no need to continue the sun-gazing practice. Some report that at this point, a person can utilize over 50 percent of their brain. If these claims hold true, the implications could be staggering.

The healthiest way to protect yourself is to…

**Drink Your Sunscreen**
While performing any sunbathing practice, using wisdom is of utmost importance. For instance, if you're a redhead with light skin, your concern about skin cancer is valid. Unfortunately, most people use sunscreen products as a solution, but they have been found to cause more harm than good. Some sunscreen products contain toxic chemicals that, when they penetrate through the skin, can increase the risk of disease… toxic chemicals such as PABA, Dioxybenzone, Oxybenzone, and Titanium Dioxide. Another major problem with sunscreen is that it blocks the skin's ability to produce vitamin D by more than 95 percent!

The answer may just be as simple as eating or drinking more fresh vegetables and berries, foods that are loaded with phytochemical-nutrients, such as antioxidants. Modern nutritional science has recently discovered new insights into how an increase of antioxidants helps to protect our skin naturally. In fact, studies on other phytochemical-nutrients, such as polyphenols and nutrients such as vitamin C, have shown that they offer protection from UVA radiation and that nutritional factors exert promising effects on the skin.

These are just a few examples...

**Foods That Protect You**
- Red, yellow, and orange fruits and veggies: These contain carotenoids, which reduce sunburn.
- Tart cherries and peppermint leaves: These contain perillyl alcohol, which stops cancer formation in human cells exposed to intense UV light.
- Leafy greens: These contain lutein and zeaxanthin, which stops UV-induced cell proliferation.
- Green tea: This contains antioxidants EGCGs, which block DNA damage in light-exposed human skin cells.
- Oranges, lemons, and limes: These contain limonene, which is linked to a 34% reduction in skin cancer.

So what are you waiting for? Why not consider drinking your sunscreen?

Try a cup of warm green tea in the morning or blend up a delectable fruit smoothie or juice a carotenoid-rich green drink. The more you drink, the greater your protection.

**Sunscreen Smoothie**
1 large orange, peeled
12 strawberries, remove stem
1 banana, peeled
1 tablespoon celery juice powder
Blend at high speed until smooth.

**Leafy Green Sunscreen**
8 stalks celery
4 kale leaves or Swiss chard
1 bunch parsley
1 handful spinach
Juice.

So go ahead! Enlighten yourself! Sunbathe your way to wellness! I did, and so can you!

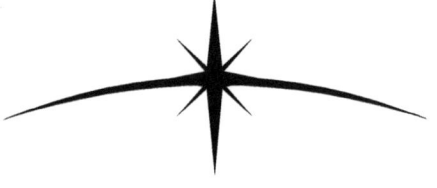

# WATER
## Drink to Enlighten Yourself

Without water, life cannot exist. Every life form that exists on Earth was conceived in and born out of water. Our bodies took form in a water sac within our mother's womb. Once the nine-month gestation period was complete, the water sac broke, and we were born—born out of water. Water is truly the gift of life.

> Earth is a water planet and so are we.

New research suggests ancient Earth began as a water world; that everything, including land, was born in and out of water, which could have major implications for the origin and evolution of life. While modern Earth's surface is about 75 percent water-covered, the new research indicates that our planet was a true ocean world some 3 billion years ago.

Interestingly, our physical bodies, like the surface of our Earth, is also 75 percent water. Every cell, like the fish in the sea, swims and bathes itself in water. Water is everywhere and flows throughout everything. We bathe in it, play in it, swim in it, get baptized in it, cook in it, and drink it.

Therefore, it's logical to conclude that every aspect of maintaining a healthy body exists within the structure of a water molecule.

When life began on Earth, streams of water flowed over rocky surfaces, causing an interaction of life forces now known as ionization. Ionization is the process of converting a molecule into an ion by adding or removing negatively charged particles such as electrons. This highly charged ionized water is characterized by groups of small cluster-size molecules that are structured and hydrogen-rich, making it possible for water to penetrate the cell membrane.

While the source of the water we drink is important, the structure of that water, being unstructured and hydrogen-poor or structured and hydrogen-rich is the most significant key.

Structured, hydrogen-rich water is characterized by groups of small cluster-size molecules called "micro-clustering" which refers to the exceptionally small "structured" molecules of water. This type of water has the profound ability to penetrate the cell membrane, enabling nutrients to easily enter and wastes to effortlessly exit.

A water molecule is like the *Holy Trinity* held within the chemistry of our physical existence—a compound of hydrogen and oxygen: 2 parts hydrogen and 1 part oxygen.

Hydrogen, which makes up 75 percent of the universe by volume, has the highest energy content per unit weight of any known fuel. Yet it never occurs by itself in nature—it always combines with other elements such as oxygen (for water) and carbon (for fossil fuel).

Unfortunately, the waters of our body, like the waters of our earth, have become unstructured and hydrogen-depleted, predisposing us to a life of suffering from various diseases that originate from dehydration.

Dehydration can even occur if you drink lots of water every day; water whose molecules are unstructured and therefore unable to penetrate through our cellular membrane and hydrate you.

To reiterate, the significance of creating smaller water molecule clusters is that, as previously stated, it makes it easier for them to penetrate the cell membrane, which enhances tissue repair, nutrient absorption, and waste removal. Smaller water clusters recreate nature's most perfect water. It is naturally oxygenated; thus it automatically increases the body's oxygen levels. Its super-hydrating micro-cluster molecules, fortified by millions of age-defying, mineralized, antioxidants, can neutralize free radicals and boost your metabolism. It also accelerates the release of harmful chemicals, heavy metals, toxic wastes, and even fat cells.

Dr. Mu Shik John, researcher and author of *The Water Puzzle and the Hexagonal Key*, states…

> "Hexagonal water, comprised of small molecular units or ring-shaped clusters, moves easily within the cellular matrix of the body, helping with nutrient absorption and waste removal. It aids metabolic processes, supports the immune system, contributes to lasting vitality and acts as a carrier of dissolved oxygen. It can provide alkaline minerals to the body, and it helps in the more efficient removal of acidic wastes. Drinking hexagonal water takes us in the direction of health. It supports long life and freedom from disease. Biological organisms prefer hexagonal water."

In essence, if water molecules are arranged in a hexagonal shape, like a honeycomb, you have what we now call hexagonal or structured water. Both waters have the same chemical makeup, but the structure causes hexagonal water to have unique properties, and healthy hydration benefits.

F. Batmanghelidj, M.D., author of Your Body's Many Cries For Water, proved in his years of research that Unintentional Chronic Dehydration (UCD) contributes to and even produces pain and many degenerative diseases that can be prevented and treated by increasing water intake on a regular basis. With the right quality and quantity of water, he believes that you can even cure the sick.

He says...

"You're not sick; you're thirsty. Don't treat thirst with medication."

Dehydration of the body is like the droughts of the earth, which occurs when a region (organs and glands) indicates a deficiency in its water supply. Thus, when you drink structured hydrogen-rich water "the rainforest way," you will no longer suffer from famines and related diseases that come from a drought!

Rainforests are forests characterized by high levels of rainfall, raining over 80 inches each year. Tropical rainforests have been called the "Jewels of the Earth" as they are havens for millions of green plants that generate much of the Earth's oxygen. In a rainforest, plants and microorganisms flourish because the rains come down in a constant mist instead of sporadic downpours. Thus, when you drink 4-6 ounces of structured hydrogen-rich water every 30 minutes every day "the rainforest way" and consume lots of fruits and greens, your inner rainforest will also flourish.

Sadly, water becomes unstructured and hydrogen-depleted, mostly caused by pollution. It has been suggested that water pollution is the leading worldwide cause of death, and that it accounts for the deaths of more than 14,000 people daily. The Centers for Disease Control and Prevention (CDC) reports that 900,000 to 1,000,000 Americans will get sick from drinking contaminated water this year alone.

They, amongst major medical journals, say that good ole' fashioned tap water can be downright lethal. It has been shown to trigger a massive heart attack, riddle your body with cancer, make your bones crumble, infect your body with deadly parasites, and much more.

The CDC reports...

> "What comes out of your faucet is not water... it's a toxic soup of chemicals, bacteria, viruses, and heavy metals!"

So, what type of water should we be drinking?

**Tap water** is the worst water you can drink (or even bathe in) because it is loaded with chemicals!

According to the Environmental Protection Agency (EPA), there are over 700 chemicals in our drinking water, and that includes "clean" sources such as wells and springs. Of all the dangerous chemicals found in drinking water, chlorine and fluoride are two of the most prominent. Other contaminants like bisphenol-A, pharmaceuticals, pesticides, bleach, industrial runoff, bacterial toxins, and toxic metals like lead, mercury, and arsenic, are some of the other things in our water that can lead to health issues, including gastrointestinal illness, reproductive problems, and neurological disorders.

**Spring water** can be healthy or unhealthy, depending on the source.

Drinking spring water can be risky. The shallower the well, the less likely bacteria and other contaminants have been filtered out of the water by rock, sand, gravel, or soil layers. Open springs also attract birds and other animals like deer, which use the spring for drinking or bathing. Chemicals from agricultural runoff are almost always found in spring waters. But if you have access to a free-running spring and it appears clean to your eyes, you can always use a filtration home system such as Berkey. Or, if you're a hiker and come across a wonderful flowing spring, there are numerous hiker filters such as Lifestraw or Sawyer squeeze that will serve your water needs well.

If you're looking for the absolute best bottled spring water, always choose Mountain Valley as they use ultra-filters to remove any naturally occurring organic matter. They also use a micron-filter to remove any microbiological particles. And best of all, they use glass instead of plastic bottles!

**Distilled water** is a type of purified water that is safe to drink, but you'll probably find it tastes bland.

When you distill water, all of the minerals are removed, along with contaminants. Water is boiled into vapor and condensed back into liquid in a separate container. Impurities in the original water that do not boil below or near the boiling point of water remain in the original container.

If you maintain a healthy and balanced diet, drinking distilled water will not leave a negative impact since you're getting vital minerals from other sources. But if you plan to drink distilled water consistently, it is important to keep up your daily intake of fruits and vegetables.

**Filtered water** is water that has been mechanically filtered or processed to remove impurities.

Filtered water does not produce that same level of purity as distilled water, but it gets very close. Depending on the type of filter, it is possible to practically eliminate contaminants while leaving helpful minerals intact. It all depends on the size of the filter and the filtration method. Carbon filters can achieve a high degree of purity with little loss of water, and they operate quite quickly. For maximum purity without distillation, though, reverse osmosis methods outcompete carbon filters. They're less efficient, but the result is great-tasting water without the odd characteristics that are often noted in distilled water.

So, what is the best hydrating water?

## Structured Hydrogen-Rich Water!

Fortunately, there's a water processing technology that creates water the way nature originally designed it to be. This water technology is called Spring Aqua.

There are several world-famous mountain springs that attract millions of people annually because of the healing properties of the water. The Netflix documentary Down to Earth features Zac Efron and Darin Olien's visit to Lourdes Springs in France.

Lourdes Springs is home to one of the most famous healing shrines in the world, it receives 4-6 million visitors a year. Many of the visitors seek cures they believe come from drinking or bathing in the water. Scientists have studied this spring water since the late 1800s hoping to unlock the mysteries and document these miraculous results.

**Spring Aqua** has developed our own version of Lourdes water through mimicking the rock layers, geology, and other properties outlined in scientific studies. As a result, they have created a complete water hydration technology that you can have right in your own home. They call it an Ecosystem in a Box and can be found on my website: tonitoney.com.

## WATER RECIPES

Drinking enough water can sometimes feel like a daunting task. We know we need to be drinking water but, let's be honest, it can be easy to forget! So, if you're like me and get bored of the tasteless taste of water, adding fruits can encourage you to drink more, simply by changing up the flavor. This helps to prevent the effects of dehydration such as constipation, mind fog, and more.

Adding fruit-flavored ingredients to your water also has health benefits, as well as tasting super good. From lemon to lime to apple to cucumber water, read on to find out more.

**Lemon Water…**
- may help with digestion.
- may potentially prevent kidney stones.
- is a good source of vitamin C.
- might help with weight loss.
- helps relieve nausea.
- helps relieve constipation.
- with ginger helps to soothe indigestion.

Instead of having a cup of coffee in the morning, how about trying a cup of warm water with the juice of one whole lemon first thing in the morning as a healthy way to start your day? Drinking warm lemon water regularly has been shown to decrease acidity in your body and remove uric acid from joints. It has also been shown to enhance enzyme function, stimulating your liver and activating bile flow, which helps emulsify and flush out fat-soluble toxins.

**Lemonade Water**
1 quart water
1 cup freshly squeezed organic lemon juice
¼ cup organic raw agave nectar or stevia
4 fresh mint sprigs

**Apple Cinnamon Water**
1 quart water
2 Fuji apples thinly shredded
4 cinnamon sticks
¼ cup organic raw agave nectar or stevia
Let sit unrefrigerated for 4-6 hours.

## WATER THERAPIES

**Detox Bath Therapy**
When you get sick with a cold or other illness, your body's natural defense is to produce a fever. With an elevated body temperature, your immune system can work at a heightened level so that your body is able to fight against any viruses or bacteria more effectively. Elevated body temperatures also increase the speed and efficiency of blood circulation, thereby increasing the supply of blood to the "battle zones" in the body while speeding the removal of toxic waste that your body is attempting to eliminate.

The higher body temperature also facilitates recovery from fatigue or stress. This is why wounded wild animals have been seen bathing in hot springs in the mountains, using their instinctual wisdom to speed up healing by soaking themselves in hot mineral water.

To take full therapeutic advantage of a detox bath, you must stay in the bath for 20 minutes or longer. While hot baths help to accelerate the detox process, when you take a Celtic Sea Salt® bath, the benefits are astounding. Not only will an enormous amount of toxins be released through the skin during the bath, but the highly charged minerals from the salt will also be absorbed, helping to remove acids and alkalinize your internal terrain. Just be sure the water you're bathing in has been filtered.

It has been noted that a person can get rid of heavy metals such as lead, mercury, arsenic, amalgam, and calcium because the whole crystal salt facilitates the breakup of their molecular structures. Saltwater therapy can also assist in releasing any calcium build-up, but for the body to get rid of these deposits, it has to first metabolize them. Even animal proteins, which are difficult to break down and eliminate, will be eliminated through the urine due to the strong structural formation of the crystal salt.

Most bath salts you'll find on store shelves, however, do not hold the cleansing and regenerating power of Celtic Bath Salts. Their crystals are truly "diamonds in the rough." Thus, for the ultimate bath, pour about two pounds of Celtic Salt Crystals into a clean, standard-sized tub. If your bathtub is not standard size, you can calculate the amount of salt required by using the formula of 1.28 ounces of salt per gallon of water. This generates a 1 percent solution.

Add just enough hot water to cover the crystals and wait for about 10 minutes, or until they have almost dissolved. Now fill the bathtub but resist the temptation to run a steaming-hot bath. Water closer to your normal body temperature, or slightly higher, will create less stress on your body. Simply fill the bathtub, keeping the water comfortably warm, but not too hot. Remain in the bath for 20-30 minutes. You may want to keep adding hot water to maintain the warm water temperature. Be sure to drink lots of water while you are bathing. If you begin to feel faint or weak, don't stay any longer; shower the salts off and towel dry.

Because the hot salt bath makes demands on the circulatory system, the process of detoxification may make you feel a little weak for a short time afterward (10-15 minutes). So, wrap yourself up in your bathrobe and enjoy relaxing as your body recovers. Note that if you have a heart condition, poor circulation, or high blood pressure, you might consider a salt footbath instead of a full bath.

**Hot and Cold-Water Therapy**
Ancient civilizations have long recognized the healing power of using alternating hot and cold water. As far back as the 4th Century, the great Greek physician Hippocrates prescribed this type of therapy for its beneficial healing effects. The Romans even built communal baths because they believed in the healing power of hot and cold applications. These alternating applications have been found to be helpful for almost every conceivable healing process known.

Hot and cold water assists better circulation of blood in the body, which helps to decrease inflammation, get more white blood cells circulating, and stimulates the white blood cells to become more effective against infection. Chronic conditions such as high blood pressure, kidney disease, diabetes, and chronic infections benefit from hot and cold hydrotherapy, which stimulates the body's immune system and improves the vital energy in the body. Acute conditions such as headaches or menstrual cramps benefit from alternating hot and cold applications to relieve pain and discomfort.

Alternating hot and cold baths are good for treating hands and feet. With water as hot as you can stand it in one bowl, ice water in the other, put hands or feet in the hot water for one minute, then plunge into the cold for 20 seconds. Then back into hot and cold again until a total of 10 minutes have been spent doing this, ending with the plunge into the ice water. This process has been reported to be beneficial for arthritic joints and tired, aching feet, plus the alternating hot and cold stimulates circulation.

An alternating hot and cold footbath is also great in promoting circulation in the legs, helping with varicose veins, insomnia, headaches, high blood pressure, as well as generating an overall sense of well-being. The best thing is… it is easily accomplished in the comfort of your own home.

**Think Good Thoughts Therapy**
Internationally renowned Japanese scientist Dr. Masaru Emoto has proven in his New York Times best-selling book, The Hidden Messages in Water, how our thoughts, words, and feelings have a profound influence on water molecules, either positively or negatively. By using high-speed photography, he discovered that crystals formed in frozen water when specific, concentrated thoughts had been directed towards it.

This was revolutionary!

He then discovered that water from clear springs, or water that had been exposed to loving words and thoughts, formed brilliant, complex, and colorful snowflake patters. In contrast, polluted springs, or water exposed to negative words and thoughts, formed incomplete, asymmetrical patterns with dull colors. The implications of this research created a new awareness of how we can positively impact the world within and all around us, for good or evil!

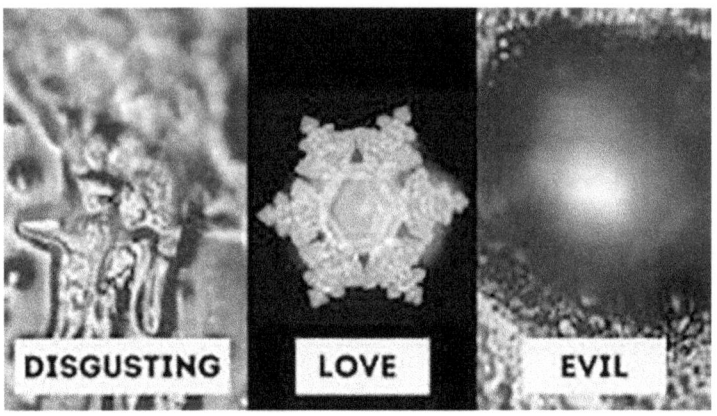

And the Lord God commanded the man...

> "You are free to eat from any tree in the garden; but you must not eat from the tree of the knowledge of good and evil, for if you do, you will surely die."
> -Genesis 2: 16-17

So how does this type of phenomena happen?

As I was contemplating this phenomenon early one morning, it occurred to me that our physical bodies are made up of chains of carbon atoms, which is why we are said to be "carbon-based life-forms." That's when it began to make more sense to my inquisitive mind! I thought about carbon paper and how when you place it between two pieces of paper, and then write on the top page, it imprints on the paper below!

Then I considered that carbon atoms are made up of 6 electrons, 6 neutrons, and 6 protons! Thus, the number... 666! Now that was an eye-opener! Could that mean that we are perhaps our own anti-Christ when we think negative thoughts about ourselves or the world around us… a mind that is in opposition to who and what we truly are?

As I was contemplating this possibility, I heard a very small still voice within me say…

> *Wherever your focus of attention goes, your chemistry flows. Likewise, wherever your focus of attention goes, your reality flows. Shift your focus of attention on what you want instead of what you don't want and watch, as the world within and all around you changes! You have nothing to do but this!*

For me, this was a profound revelation!

Consider the Cherokee story of…

## THE TWO WOLVES

A young boy came to his grandfather, filled with anger at another boy who had done him an injustice.

The old grandfather said to his grandson…

> "Let me tell you a story. I too, at times, have felt a great hate for those that have taken so much, with no sorrow for what they do. But hate wears you down, and hate does not hurt your enemy. Hate is like taking poison and wishing your enemy would die. I have struggled with these feelings many times.

It is as though there are two wolves inside me; one wolf is good and does no harm. He lives in harmony with all around him and does not take offence when no offence was intended. He will only fight when it is right to do so, and in the right way. But the other wolf, is full of anger. The littlest thing will set him into a fit of temper.

He fights everyone, all the time, for no reason. He cannot think because his anger and hate are so great. It is helpless anger, because his anger will change nothing. Sometimes it is hard to live with these two wolves inside me, because both of the wolves try to dominate my spirit."

The boy looked intently into his grandfather's eyes and asked, "So which wolf will win, grandfather?"

The Grandfather smiled and said, "The one I feed."

So go ahead! Enlighten yourself! Think your way to wellness! I did, and so can you!

Following The Four "Fuel" Groups is simple and easy. Better yet, it's a great way to build that strong foundation toward becoming the healthy, happier, more ENLIGHTENED YOU that you were designed to be. Just know that when you start aligning yourself with the four elemental forces of nature—earth, air, fire, and water—the enlightening process is steady but sure. And all you have to do to begin the journey to that healthier, happier, more ENLIGHTENED YOU is to start by enjoying the journey back home again to your true self!

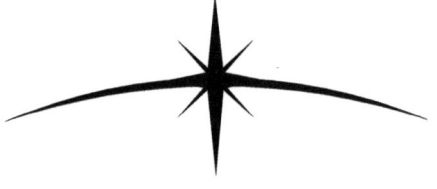

# ADDENDUM

## FOOD HAS ESSENTIAL PRINCIPLES

After being in the nutritional field for over 30 years, I have come to believe that food has essentials principles, as do the trillions of cells that swim throughout our body's watery terrain! The following essential food principles are what I personally follow that helps me sustain a state of perfect health.

## ESSENTIAL FOOD PRINCIPLE #1
## Consume Whole, Organic Plant Foods Only

This principle is to consume a diet of whole, organic plant foods only. This principle emphasizes a deep connection between what we eat and how it impacts not only our physical health but also our overall life energy. The idea of consuming a diet of whole, organic plant foods align with both ancient wisdom and modern nutritional science.

The phrase "the whole is greater than the sum of its parts" is central to this philosophy. Whole, organic plant foods contain a synergy of nutrients, enzymes, and other bioactive compounds that work together to promote health in ways that isolated nutrients cannot. For example, eating an apple with its skin provides fiber, antioxidants, and other protective nutrients in a balanced way, unlike consuming a single nutrient in a supplement form.

Here's why this principle is so essential:

**Oxygenation and Alkalization:** Whole, organic plant foods are known for their ability to support an alkaline environment in the body. An alkaline body is believed to reduce inflammation, increase vitality, and optimize cellular function. Plant foods, especially greens, fruits, and vegetables, are rich in oxygen-boosting chlorophyll, which helps to revitalize the blood and tissues.

**Connection to Nature:** There's something spiritually rejuvenating about eating food that is natural, whole, and untouched by artificial chemicals. It's a return to our roots, supporting both physical and spiritual well-being. By focusing on seed-bearing plants, you're aligning with the principle of Genesis—a return to eating what was originally intended for us.

**A Shift in Consciousness:** Eating a whole food, plant-based diet requires a shift in how we view food. It's not just about sustenance; it's about nourishment on a deeper level. The principle asks for more than just a dietary change—it calls for a shift in lifestyle, mindset, and awareness. Preparing meals from scratch, understanding the sourcing of your food, and creating meals that are vibrant and full of life is a profound act of self-care.

**Practical Application:** As you move towards consuming more whole, organic plant foods, you'll find that it's not only about adding more fruits and vegetables but also exploring new flavors, textures, and cuisines. The variety of plant foods available today makes the transition both exciting and fulfilling. Nuts and seeds, for example, offer healthy fats and protein, balancing out the meal in a nourishing way.

This principle sets the foundation for an entirely new way of thinking about food—one that promotes vitality, harmony, and connection. The emphasis on organic foods also suggests an awareness of sustainability and the impact of our choices on the planet. This holistic approach is about becoming your best self through your food choices.

So, how do you envision incorporating this principle into your life?

## ESSENTIAL FOOD PRINCIPLE #2
## Consume Lots of Raw, Living Plant Foods

Eating a diet high in raw, living plant foods is the highest and best way to prepare your physical body for the shift of the ages. If 75 to 100 percent of your total food consumption consists of raw, living foods, you are considered what some call a New Earth "raw foodist." This simply means that most of the foods you're eating are in their natural, raw, whole-food, organic state—foods that are unprocessed and mostly uncooked. The greater the percentage of raw, living food in your diet, the greater the electrical energy in and around every cell of your body!

Raw foods are considered "living" foods because they contain life energy producing enzymes. Enzymes are a long string of amino acids that exists in every living thing that makes normal cellular function possible. They act as a catalyst for chemical reactions in cells, which means that they either initiate or speed up chemical processes. Many chemical processes require high speed to react appropriately, so you could look at enzymes as life supporting engines of cellular chemical reactions.

Enzymes are responsible for initiating the digestion of foods, which is the primary reason that raw foods are so valuable to the body. In essence, raw foods bring their own enzymes to the party, making it easier for our bodies to digest them. This is not the case with cooked foods.

This is where raw, living foods play a very significant role. Enzymes are very sensitive to heat above 118°F. When food is cooked, steamed, canned, pasteurized, baked, or boiled above 120°F, it loses virtually all its enzyme activity. So, in the process of digestion, the body must borrow enzymes from the body rather than from the food itself, resulting in a drain on our system. This is why you may feel sluggish after eating a cooked meal.

Eating raw, living foods can also support detoxification, giving the body more energy for healing, growth, and optimal function. Many raw food advocates believe this lifestyle helps promote clarity of mind, improved digestion, and a higher sense of vitality.

Food for Thought: For a caterpillar to transform into a butterfly, it digests itself using enzymes triggered by hormones!

## HOW TO INCORPORATE RAW, LIVING FOODS

**Start with Smoothies & Juices:** Blending fruits and vegetables is an easy way to consume a wide range of raw, living foods in one meal. Including seeds, skin (where possible), and even peels can help you maximize the nutritional benefits.

**Raw Salads and Wraps:** You can create a variety of fresh, nutritious salads with leafy greens, sprouts, seeds, nuts, and raw vegetables. Use dressings made from raw ingredients like olive oil, lemon, and avocado.

**Snacking on Fresh Produce:** Having fresh fruits and vegetables on hand as snacks is an easy way to increase your raw food intake. Carrot sticks, cucumber slices, or raw nuts can satisfy hunger while giving your body a boost of nutrients.

**Cultured Foods:** Incorporating raw, cultured foods like nuts and seeds can further enhance your gut health with live probiotics, enzymes, and additional phytochemicals.

**Raw Sprouts and Seeds:** Sprouts like broccoli, mung beans, and sunflower are nutrient-dense, and seeds (such as chia, flax, and hemp) offer healthy fats and proteins in their raw form.

## ESSENTIAL FOOD PRINCIPLE #3
## Consume Organic Produce Only

This principle of always choosing organic produce goes beyond simply supporting a more natural or eco-friendly approach to farming—it's about choosing foods that sustain both our health and the planet's. The contrast between organic and conventionally grown produce is stark, especially when considering the health implications, environmental impact, and long-term sustainability.

Here's a breakdown of the key points:

### Toxins and Health

Pesticides and Herbicides: Conventionally grown crops often carry toxic residues from synthetic pesticides, herbicides, and fertilizers. Over time, these chemicals accumulate in the body, contributing to health issues like hormonal disruption, cancer, neurological problems, and more. For sensitive individuals, even low levels of exposure can result in immediate symptoms, such as headaches, dizziness, skin reactions, or digestive disturbances.

### Organic Foods and Health

Organic farming avoids synthetic pesticides and fertilizers. Organic farmers use natural methods, such as composting and crop rotation, to enrich the soil and promote healthy, vibrant plant life. This results in foods that are not only free of harmful chemicals but also richer in essential nutrients. Organic foods are found to have higher levels of antioxidants, vitamins, and minerals compared to their conventionally grown counterparts.

### Nutrient Density

The nutritional differences between organic and conventional produce are not just theoretical — studies suggest that organic foods tend to have higher concentrations of vitamins, minerals, and antioxidants. This makes organic foods a better choice for anyone looking to maximize their intake of nutrients and support overall health. Nutrient-dense foods also help our bodies resist illness and maintain optimal energy levels.

## Ecological Impact

One of the major differences between organic and conventional farming is how they treat the soil. Conventional farming, with its reliance on synthetic chemicals, tends to deplete the soil of its natural fertility and microorganisms, causing long-term environmental damage. Organic farming, on the other hand, nurtures the soil through composting, crop rotation, and reduced chemical input, maintaining a healthier, more sustainable ecosystem.

## Genetically Modified Organisms (GMOs)

Conventional farming frequently uses genetically engineered seeds to increase yield or resistance to pests. These seeds can alter the genetic makeup of crops and potentially cause unknown long-term effects on both human health and biodiversity. Organic farming, by definition, avoids GMOs, supporting biodiversity and ecological balance.

## Visual Evidence

The book *The Invisible Power Within Foods* by Walter Danzer offers a fascinating look at the difference between organic and conventional produce under magnification. The tissues of organic foods show clear, well-organized structural integrity, while conventional foods display incoherence and signs of ecological breakdown. This can serve as a visual metaphor for the broader differences in health and vitality between the two types of farming systems.

## The Accumulation of Exposure

Most people don't realize that consuming conventionally grown produce regularly leads to an accumulation of toxic chemicals in the body. Over time, this buildup can contribute to chronic health problems that may seem unrelated to diet. By choosing organic, you are reducing your body's exposure to these chemicals, protecting your health in the long run.

Always choosing organic food is not just about avoiding harmful chemicals— it's about embracing a more holistic and conscious way of nourishing the body. When you choose organic, you're opting for food that is not only better for your body but also better for the planet. You're supporting agricultural practices that maintain ecological balance, foster biodiversity, and reduce the negative environmental footprint of farming.

This principle encourages you to think more deeply about where your food comes from and how it impacts your body and the world around you. It's a call to choose quality over convenience, sustainability over exploitation, and health over short-term cost savings.

Incorporating this principle into your life can be as simple as making a habit of shopping at local farmers' markets, selecting organic items at your regular grocery store, or even growing your own organic garden if you have the space and interest.

## ESSENTIAL FOOD PRINCIPLE #4
### Consume Locally Grown, Seasonal Foods

This principle is about why choosing locally and seasonally grown produce is so essential. Foods grown close to home are saturated with an abundance of phytochemical- nutrition because it is picked close to its ripened peak.

Eating locally and seasonally can also be healthy for the environment. Buying foods purchased from your "food shed," loosely defined as farms within 100 miles of your home, helps to curtail the issue with carbon and global warming.

Shipping and trucking food from every corner of the world requires millions of gallons of gasoline for transportation, not to mention all the pollution it releases into the environment, just getting to the supermarket. Produce purchased from the supermarket has been picked unripen then shipped in cold refiguration for days or even weeks, whereas produce purchased from a local farmer's market has often been picked within 24 hours of your purchase. This freshness not only affects the flavor of your food, but the nutritional value as well, which declines with time and changes in temperature.

Spending your money at a local farmer's market not only supports your health and the environment, but it also supports the livelihood of farmers in your community as well as the local economy. Eat Seasonal Foods Seasonal eating is a sustainable way of eating that has numerous health advantages.

This lifestyle encourages you to only eat fruits and vegetables that are in season for your geographic area, such as eating pears in the fall, oranges in the winter, asparagus in the spring, tomatoes in the summer, and so on. Seasonal foods are fresher, tastier and more nutritious than food consumed out of season.

Even though we all like to eat strawberries or watermelon year-round, the best time to eat them is when they can be purchased directly from a local grower shortly after harvest.

As you know, for those of us who do not live in the tropics, there are four growing and harvesting seasons:

**Spring, Summer, Fall, and Winter.** Each season brings its own bounty, and consuming food that aligns with the natural cycles of your environment is not only healthier but also more aligned with sustainability.

This summary of seasonal foods is beautifully aligned with the natural cycles of the year. Eating seasonally not only helps with maintaining a balanced diet but also connects us more deeply with the rhythms of the environment around us. Here's a more refined way to think about these foods by season:

## SPRINGTIME EATING

Springtime offers light, refreshing, and detoxifying foods that help cleanse the body after the heavier meals of winter. These foods are high in water content, antioxidants, and vitamins, especially vitamin C, which supports the immune system as the weather warms up.

### Springtime Foods

| | | |
|---|---|---|
| Leafy greens | Asparagus | Cherries |
| Culinary herbs | Artichokes | Pineapple |
| Avocadoes | Peas | Lemon |
| Spring onions | Rhubarb | Apricots |
| Radishes | Strawberries | |

# SUMMERTIME EATING

Summertime foods are vibrant, sweet, and hydrating. They help keep the body cool and energized during the heat. Fruits and vegetables are at their juiciest and often contain high amounts of vitamins A, C, and potassium, supporting hydration, skin health, and overall vitality.

## Summertime Foods

| | | |
|---|---|---|
| Tomatoes | Eggplant | Peaches |
| Cucumbers | Okra | Nectarines |
| Zucchini | Green beans | Cherries |
| Peppers | Corn | Mangoes |
| Cucumber | Melons | Papaya |
| Summer squash | Berries | |

# AUTUMTIME EATING

As the weather cools, autumntime foods become heartier and more grounding. Root vegetables and squash provide comfort, with complex carbohydrates and fiber to keep you nourished and stable. The rich colors of these foods, from deep orange to vibrant red, also signal the abundance of antioxidants and vitamins like beta-carotene, which support immune health.

## Autumntime Foods

| | | |
|---|---|---|
| Pumpkins | Squashes | Cauliflower |
| Sweet potatoes | Brussels sprouts | Cabbage |

| | | |
|---|---|---|
| Kale | Figs | Plums |
| Lettuce | Apples | Raspberries |
| Broccoli | Grapes | Cranberries |
| Beets | Blackberries | Persimmons |
| Carrots | Pears | |

## WINTERTIME EATING

Wintertime foods are dense and nourishing, rich in nutrients to support immunity and help the body withstand cold temperatures. Citrus fruits provide a boost of vitamin C, while hearty root vegetables and cabbages offer fiber, vitamins, and minerals to maintain strength and warmth.

### Wintertime Foods

| | | |
|---|---|---|
| Root vegetables | Squashes | Apples |
| Cabbages | Radishes | Pears |
| Kale | Chard | Kiwi |
| Collard greens | Chestnuts | Pomegranates |
| Leeks | Citrus fruits | Persimmons |

By consuming foods that are in season, we not only help our bodies adapt to the changing weather but also support sustainability by reducing the carbon footprint associated with transporting out-of-season produce. Eating in harmony with nature's cycles is not only nourishing but also eco-friendly!

## The Benefits of Eating Seasonally:

Nutritional Value: Seasonal produce is typically harvested at its peak of ripeness, ensuring it's packed with more nutrients, vitamins, and minerals than out-of-season counterparts that are picked prematurely.

- Better Taste: When fruits and vegetables are consumed in season, they often taste better—sweeter, juicier, and more flavorful—because they're allowed to fully ripen before harvesting.

- Environmental Impact: Local and seasonal eating reduces the carbon footprint. It requires less energy for transportation, refrigeration, and storage, helping mitigate the effects of global warming and environmental degradation.

- Cost-Effective: Seasonal foods tend to be more affordable because they are abundant in that time of year, reducing the need for expensive storage or transportation.

- Supports Local Economies: When you buy local, you›re directly contributing to the well-being of your community. Supporting local farmers and markets ensures that these small businesses can thrive, and it keeps your money within your local economy.

This principle outlines the fact that eating locally and seasonally doesn't just mean eating fresh and nutritious food—it also allows you to reconnect with the natural rhythms of your environment and supports a more sustainable, mindful approach to food.

# ESSENTIAL FOOD PRINCIPLE #5
# Consume the Right Type of Salt, Oil, and Sugar

When you eat the wrong type of salt, oil, and sugar, your body will eventually send you and SOS (salt-oil-sugar) signal to warn you of a potential ecological threat! Here's a summary of the key points:

> **SALT: The Wrong Type**—Refined salt, often called "white poison," is heavily processed, containing mostly sodium chloride along with harmful chemicals like moisture absorbents, anti-caking agents, and synthetic iodine and fluorine. These additives can be harmful, contributing to health risks such as high blood pressure, heart disease, and cancer.
>
> **The Right Type**—Whole food sea salt, such as Celtic Sea Salt, is natural, unrefined, and rich in electrolytes and essential trace minerals. This salt supports the body's pH, natural electrolyte balance, and overall vitality. It is harvested traditionally, preserving its natural state and life-giving properties.
>
> **OIL: The Wrong Type**—Processed vegetable oils, especially seed oils like canola, corn, soybean, and cottonseed oils, are high in oxidized omega-6 fatty acids. These oils contribute to inflammation, cell damage, and various chronic diseases, including metabolic disorders and macular degeneration.
>
> **The Right Type**—Organic, cold-pressed olive oil rich in polyphenols (antioxidants) is the healthiest choice. Olive oil from regions like Crete and Morocco, especially when the

olives are harvested early, has the highest levels of polyphenols. While olive oil is beneficial, it should be used sparingly since oils are concentrated fats.

**SUGAR: The Wrong Type**—Refined sugar, stripped of its naturally occurring minerals and nutrients, has been linked to a range of health issues, including obesity, insulin resistance, heart disease, and even depression and cancer. Even though sugar from honey may be organic, raw, and harvested with the highest sustainable practices, it still creates an abnormal insulin spike. Honey is not a plant-based product, and therefore, goes against our New Earth whole food, plant-based diet principles.

**The Right Type**—Whole food natural sugars are found in fruits and various other plant-based, vegan sugars such as organic raw agave or coconut nectar, which have a low glycemic index. These plant-based sugars come with beneficial nutrients, fiber, vitamins, and minerals that make them much healthier for the body than refined sugar. Whole fruits, in particular, are not the enemy; it's the combination of fruits with the wrong fats that can cause issues.

**Key Takeaway**
Focus on consuming unrefined, whole foods—like natural salts, high-quality oils, and unrefined sugars—instead of their processed counterparts. These support your body's natural systems, enhance vitality, and prevent chronic diseases. This principle reinforces the idea that food in its purest, least altered form is the most nourishing for the body.

# ESSENTIAL FOOD PRINCIPLE #6
## Proper Food Combining

This principle is to properly combine the types of foods you eat. While certain food-combining principles are as ancient as the Mosaic Covenant (the Jewish law requiring the separating of meat and dairy), some of today's top nutritional researchers report that some foods are digested differently, thus should be eaten separately and at different times. There are plenty of books on the subject, and I recommend reading up on this practice, especially if you have issues with digestion.

Fruits and non-starchy vegetables are digested quickly and easily. Other foods require more time and specialized enzymatic functions. The most important rule is to separate a meal of carbohydrate-rich foods such as rice, bananas and carrots from protein-rich foods such as beans, nuts and seeds.

According to the studies of Dr. Herbert M. Shelton, one of the greatest natural hygienists and the father of food combining, there are sound physiological reasons for eating, separately, foods that require different digestive enzymes and gastric juices in the mouth, stomach and small intestines.

Starchy foods, such as potatoes, require an alkaline digestive medium, which is supplied initially in the mouth by the enzyme ptyalin.

Protein foods require an acid medium for digestion, which is supplied in the stomach by acid enzymes and hydrochloric acid.

Hydrochloric acid destroys ptyalin and suspends the digestion of starches. Undigested starch in the stomach interferes with the digestion of protein. It absorbs and neutralizes the enzyme pepsin, which is required for the digestion of protein.

In short, acid and alkaline digestive mediums neutralize each other. Therefore, if you eat a starch food with a protein food, digestion may be impaired or completely arrested. These undigested foods can cause various kinds of digestive disorders.

Another newly discovered, food-combining rule: Never combine fruits with fats!

Most vegans, vegetarians and even raw foodists are consuming way too many fats in their diets in the form of nuts, seeds and oils. The problem arises when a high-fat diet is combined with a high-fruit diet. Ultimately, fruits and fats do not mix! When eaten together, they can create a health-debilitating perfect storm.

Dr. Neal Barnard, in his book, *How to Reverse Diabetes*, scientifically proved that, over time, undigested fats can accumulate around the membrane (skin) of our cells, which inhibits insulin's ability to carry glucose into the cells to be converted into energy and out of the bloodstream. If glucose is allowed to build up in our bloodstream, everything from insulin resistance to type-2 diabetes can occur. Even Candida can grow out of control in its attempt to consume the sugar.

Therefore, the more fat you eat when consuming a high fruit, high carbohydrate diet, the less effective insulin is at getting glucose into the cells and out of the bloodstream; this is why, a high fat, high protein diet works, such as Keto and Paleo. No sugar, no problem; you can lose weight because there's not a build-up of glucose in the blood stream!

However, when consuming this type of unnatural diet long term, they might just eventually create unnatural side-effects, such as acidosis.

So, how about a more natural alkaline diet, a diet that nature intended for us! That means, a diet of carbohydate foods such as fruit! But remember, when you eat fruit, NEVER eat fat, like nuts or avocadoes, at the same time!

It's as simple as that!

## ESSENTIAL FOOD PRINCIPLE #7
## Follow Nature's Circadian Rhythm

This principle is focused on following certain daily cycles known as the circadian rhythm. Circadian refers to the regular recurrence of cycles of activity that occur approximately every 24 hours, or one full day. The rhythm is linked to the sun and the moon's light- dark cycle. While sleep cycles are the most common studied by science, it has also been found that if one's daily eating patterns are in tune with these naturally occurring rhythms, people notice a tremendous increase in their overall health, energy and well-being.

According to natural hygienists, there are three cycles associated with the circadian rhythm: (1) consumption (eating and digesting); (2) assimilation (extracting nutrients and assimilating); and (3) elimination (purging and releasing). Each has its own eight-hour period during which its activities are the most heightened.

*The consumption cycle* is from noon until 8 pm. This is the time when the body is most capable of efficiently taking in and digesting food.

*The assimilation cycle* is from 8 pm until 4 am. This is the time the body is extracting nutrients and assimilating what it needs.

*The elimination cycle* is from 4 am until noon. This is the time when the body is gathering wastes and preparing them for elimination.

## Step 1: The Consumption Cycle

Food should be eaten between noon and 8 pm. This is when your body is in the consumption cycle. The consumption cycle occurs when the body is predisposed to eating and digesting food and allotting the energy to do so. Chinese medicine has long taught that our digestive fire increases and decreases according to the position of the sun. Thus, because the sun is at its highest and greatest intensity from noon until 3 pm, these three hours, according to this tradition, are the most optimal time to consume the majority of our food.

## Step 2: The Assimilation Cycle

Food should not be eaten between 8 pm and 4 am. This is when your body switches from the consumption cycle to the assimilation cycle and starts the process of extracting and assimilating the nutrients from the food you've eaten during the consumption cycle. Hence, after the food you've consumed has been digested, energy is needed to extract and utilize the nutrients the body requires for optimal function. If food is eaten after 8 pm, your body is forced out of the assimilation cycle and back into the consumption cycle, diverting energy away from proper nutrient extraction and uptake and stressing your digestive system.

## Step 3: The Elimination Cycle
Food should not be eaten between 4 am to noon. This is when your body is in the elimination cycle. Food consumed prior to the completion of the elimination cycle not only severely retards the process of eliminating the accumulated wastes from the body, but it also throws the rhythm of the three cycles into turmoil. The best way to flush out the accumulated waste during this cycle is to drink 16 to 32 ounces of purified, structured water upon waking.

Then, if you feel the need to eat, consume fruit only until noon as fruits require very little digestive energy. They also hold the plant kingdom's honor of being nature's greatest food for cleansing waste from the physical body. But if you can, no calories at all until noon, even from fruits. Then break the fasting elimination cycle around noon... breakfast... with lots of seasonal fruits! Your body will be glad you did!

## The Power of Undereating
Interestingly, science has recently validated the transformational power of following Nature's Circadian Rhythms. However, they call it, intermittent fasting.

Studying a range of organisms, from yeast and roundworms to rodents and monkeys, intermittent fasting researchers found that their maximum life span could be increased up to 50 percent, simply by underfeeding and intermittently fasting them.

Researchers discovered that undereating reduces the incidence of neurological disease, age- related cancer, cardiovascular disease, and immune deficiencies in rodents, while a high-calorie intake or overfeeding increased the risk for all degenerative diseases, such as cardiovascular disease, various types of cancers, type-2 diabetes, and stroke.

Undereating was also shown to have a positive effect on brain function and debilitating diseases such as Alzheimer's, Parkinson's and strokes.

Undereating seems to protect neurons (a cell that transmits nerve impulses) against degeneration and stimulates the production of new neurons from stem cells, which may increase the ability of the brain to resist aging and restore function after an injury. While vitamins, minerals and antioxidants may improve the health of the brain, it was shown that the major factor for brain health is undereating and an increase in the time between meals.

Researchers at the University of California, Berkeley, showed that healthy mice, given only 5 percent fewer calories than mice allowed to eat freely, experienced a significant reduction in cell proliferation in several tissues, considered an indicator for cancer risk. However, mice that ate less calories instead of just reducing food intake, lived a longer, healthier life.

Cell proliferation is the increase in cellular division that takes place just before genetic repair is made, and cancer is essentially the uncontrolled division of cells. It was discovered that a cell will try to fix any damage that has occurred to its DNA, but if it divides before it has a chance to fix the damage, then that damage passes on to the offspring cells. Slowing down the rate of cell proliferation essentially buys time for the cells to repair genetic damage. This was, indeed, very significant research!

Substantial calorie reduction (up to 50 percent in some studies), not only reduces the rate of cell proliferation, but it can extend maximum life span from 30 to 70 percent of a variety of organisms, including rats, flies, worms, and yeast. It was found that mice on a 33 percent reduced calorie diet exhibited significantly decreased cell proliferation rates for skin, breast and T (lymphocyte) cells.

The greatest effect was seen after one month on the regimen, when proliferation of skin cells registered only 61 percent of that for mice fed freely. The surprising finding came with the results of the more modest 5 percent reduced calorie diet that was fed intermittently. Mice in this group had skin cell division rates that were 81 percent of those for mice fed freely.

So even just a small reduction in calories makes a big difference in terms of your body's healing power.

Researchers discovered that fasting every other day also decreased the chance of breast cancer. In all cases, division rates for breast cells were reduced the most. Mice with the lowest calorie diet had breast cell proliferation results that were only 11 percent of those in the controlled group; mice fed intermittently had results that were 37 percent of those in the controlled group.

Undereating, along with intermittent fasting, was also found to enhance insulin sensitivity and lower risk of heart disease.

### The Problem

We're overtaxing our digestive systems by not following nature's circadian rhythms. Our bodies need time to digest, assimilate and eliminate waste. If waste is allowed to accumulate, our "inner seas" become toxic and acidic, which sets up a breeding ground for reducer organisms, such as viruses, bacteria, candida, and fungus to overgrow in their attempt to clean up the toxic mess. Reducer organisms are like roaches that show up in kitchens where there's left over food particles. In essence, "if ya feed 'em, they're going to come!"

**The Solution**
Stop feeding them! Eat less and fast often on easily digestible organic fruits and vegetables. These "fast exit foods," along with intermittent fasting, gives your body the time it needs to "clean house!" When your internal environment is "swept free" of toxic wastes, your body will be functioning at peak performance.

**But what if I get hungry between meals?**
Over the years, our bodies have adapted to eating three "square" meals a day. However, if you feel hungry, try feeding your skin with a little sunlight! Melatonin, triggered by darkness, can also trigger the sensation of hunger; and low levels of vitamin D levels, triggered by a lack of sunlight, can also trigger fat storage.

So, if you're sick and tired, overweight and always hungry, simply go outside and expose your skin to the early morning rays of the sun. That means, if you eat light, you'll become light!

# FINDING IT CHALLENGING TO SHIFT?

Ah, yes. Old habits and emotional eating are such powerful forces.

Even when we know better, it's so easy to fall back into familiar routines or use food as a source of comfort. I think a lot of people, even with the best intentions, struggle with these because food is not just about nutrition—it's deeply connected to our emotions, memories, and even our sense of identity. Here are a few ways those two challenges tend to manifest:

**Old Habits**
We're creatures of habit, and the way we eat often becomes ingrained in us over years—sometimes even decades. Whether it's a diet of processed foods, comfort foods, or simply the tendency to skip meals or overeat, these habits feel automatic. The body becomes conditioned to crave the same foods, and it can be hard to break out of those cycles, even when we know they're not serving us well.

When you've been eating a certain way for years, the taste, texture, and even the rituals around food can feel comforting or "normal," and the idea of making a drastic change can be overwhelming. The difficulty often comes from retraining the brain and the body to crave something different—something healthier. It's not just a matter of willpower; it's about rewiring neural pathways and establishing new, positive associations with food that take time.

**Emotional Eating**
Emotional eating is even trickier because it's often subconscious. Many of us turn to food for comfort, stress relief, or to fill emotional voids—whether it's dealing with sadness, boredom, loneliness, anxiety, or even celebrations. Food becomes a coping mechanism, and it can feel like the only way to soothe ourselves in tough moments.

The problem with emotional eating is that it often brings short-term relief but doesn't address the underlying issue. So, you end up reaching for comfort foods, but it doesn't solve whatever emotional trigger led you to eat in the first place. Over time, emotional eating can cause guilt, self-criticism, and reinforce unhealthy food habits.

**The Overlap Between Both**
The challenging part is that old habits and emotional eating often overlap. The more we reach for food to cope with emotions, the more those eating patterns become entrenched as habits. It's a vicious cycle where emotional comfort and food become intertwined, making it hard to untangle and change.

**Breaking the Challenges**
Breaking these cycles requires more than just willpower; it requires changing your relationship with food and learning to nourish both the body and the mind. Here are some strategies that might help:

> **Mindful Eating**
> This can be a game-changer because it encourages you to eat slowly, savor your food, and tune into how you feel both physically and emotionally while eating. It's about reconnecting with your body's natural hunger cues and learning to eat for nourishment rather than emotional relief.
>
> **Emotional Awareness**
> Instead of using food to numb feelings, becoming more aware of your emotions can help you address them more directly. Journaling, talking with a friend, or even practicing mindfulness can create space between the emotion and the reaction, giving

you a chance to choose a healthier coping mechanism.

**Small, Sustainable Changes**
Rather than completely overhauling your diet overnight, start with small, achievable changes. This could mean swapping out one processed snack for some fruit or incorporating one more vegetable into your meal each day. These incremental steps can add up to big changes without feeling overwhelming.

**Replace Comfort Foods with Healthier Versions**
Emotional eating often revolves around certain comfort foods—think sweets, salty snacks, or fried foods. Finding healthier alternatives that still provide comfort, like roasted sweet potatoes, homemade energy bars, or a warm bowl of vegetable soup, can help satisfy the craving without derailing your progress.

**Exercise and Stress Relief**
Exercise is not only great for the body, but it also helps manage stress and improve mood. It can be a great way to release pent-up emotions and reduce the urge to turn to food for emotional comfort.

**Support System**
Having someone—whether a friend, family member, or even a health coach or therapist—who understands the challenges of breaking old habits can be incredibly motivating. They can offer encouragement, advice, or simply a listening ear when you need it.

**The Reward of Shifting Mindsets**

It's not an easy journey, but by recognizing the emotional and habitual patterns behind what we eat, we can begin to consciously shift those behaviors over time. The rewards aren't just physical—feeling energized, lighter, and more balanced—but emotional as well.

There's a certain empowerment that comes from realizing that you don't need to use food to handle your emotions, and that by giving your body the nutrition it craves, you're truly taking care of yourself from the inside out.

So… if you're ready, let the SHIFT begin!

# THE NEW EARTH VISION

As I closed my eyes, I saw...

> An earth within the earth—like a universe within the universe. This New Earth is emerging. Its waters are holy, streaming through towns and cities, and when we drink of this living water, we never die. For it holds the eternal code of life.
>
> It's a place without suffering—a place where the tree of life offers us its fruit—a place where the air is celestial; the light eternal; the day without
> night. It's a place where people love each other as themselves—a place that could only be called Heaven on Earth.
>
> Our physical bodies must be made ready, for in this vibrant new world, fear and death have lost their hold. And in the twinkling of an eye, our mortal bodies will become a body of light. The body that once died will now forever live.
>
> Blessed are you who are prepared to enter. Only one question remains is... are you ready?

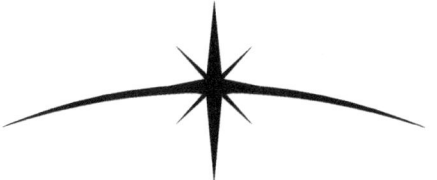

# REFERENCE NOTES

## PART ONE – THE FALL

### CHAPTER 1: THE ILLUSION OF SEPARATION

For The Medical Philosophy of Hippocrates (460–377 BCE), see Ann Wigmore, *The Hippocrates Diet and Health Program: A Natural Diet and Health Program for Weight Control, Disease Prevention, and Life Extension* (New York: Avery Trade, 1983).

Nancy Appleton, *The Curse of Louis Pasteur: Why Medicine Is Not Healing a Diseased World* (Santa Monica: Choice Publishing, 1999). A portrait of the lives of Béchamp and Pasteur and their contrasting theories.

Christopher Bird, "To Be or Not to Be? 150 Years of Hidden Knowledge," *Nexus Magazine,* April 1992. An introduction to the internal terrain theory and the amazing habits of microzymas.

"Biological Terrain vs. the Germ Theory," The Health Advantage, http://thehealthadvantage.com/ biologicalterrain.html

Antoine Béchamp, *The Third Element of the Blood,* trans Montague R Leverson (1911; Collingwood, Vic: Zigguart, 1994).

Better Living Through Chemistry? https://www.theguardian.com/environment/2024/jan/04/the-race-to-destroy-the-toxic-forever-chemicals-polluting-our-world

Pollution is Destroying Our Earth: https://sentientmedia.org/humans-destroying-ecosystems/

Pollution is Baby's Umbilical Cords: https://www.ewg.org/research/body-burden-pollution-newborns#:~:text=Tests%20revealed%20a%20total%20of,coal%2C%20gasoline%2C%20and%20garbage

Albert Einstein Quote: https://www.la.utexas.edu/users/bump/DassEinstein.pdf

## CHAPTER 2: OUR BODY OUR EARTH

Your Elemental Composition: Derived from H. A. Harper, V. W. Rodwell, P.A. Mayes, Review of Physiological Chemistry, 16th ed. (Los Altos, CA: Lange Medical Publications, 1977).

Deanna M Minich, Ph.D., FACN, CNS, Jeffrey S Bland, Ph.D., FACN, "Acid-Alkaline Balance: Role in Chronic Disease and Detoxification," *Alternative Therapies* 13, no 4 (2007).

Albert Einstein, letter of 1950, as quoted in *The New York Times* (March 29, 1972) and *The New York Post* (Nov 28, 1972).

Unnatural Feeding: Peter Montague, "Pollution of World's Largest Lakes Shows Importance of Banning Toxics," Environmental Research Foundation publication 146 (1989), www.rachel. org

Candida and Algae: Doug Jeanneret, "Lake Erie Water Quality: Past, Present and Future," Fact Sheet 046 (Columbus, OH: Ohio Sea Grant College Program, 1989), http://www.sg.ohio- state.edu/ publications/water/fs-046.html

Spencer Hunt, "Algae, Invaders Threaten Lake Erie," *The Columbus Dispatch,* Nov 25, 2012, http://www.dispatch.com/ content/stories/local/2012/11/25/algae- invaders-threaten-lake- erie.html

Martha M. Grout, M.D., (H), "Inflammation," Arizona Center for Advanced Medicine, 2007, http:// www.arizonaadvancedmedicine.com/articles/inflammation. html

USA Today Toledo, Ohio Article, http://www.usatoday.com/ story/news/nation/2014/08/03/toledo-toxins-water/13539145/

Candida: Nature's Clean-Up Crew: Josep Guarro, Josepa Gené, and Alberto M Stchigel, "Developments in Fungal Taxonomy," *Clin Microbiol Rev* 12, no 3 ( July 1999): 454–500.

Candida Yeast Infection Self Exams, National Candida Center, http:// www. nationalCandidacenter.com/Candida-self-exams/

Diabetes: The Cause, The Cure: Douglas N Graham, D.C., *The 80/10/10 Diet* (Key Largo, FL: FoodnSport Press, 2006), p. 38.

Neal D Barnard, M.D., *Neal Barnard's Program for Reversing Diabetes* (New York: Rodale, 2007).

Patrick Schrauwen, "High Fat Diet, Muscular Lipotoxicity and Insulin Resistance," *Proceedings of the Nutrition Society* 66 (2007), 33–41, doi: 10.1017/ S0029665107005277

John McDougall, M.D., interview by Dennis Hughes, http:// www.shareguide.com/ McDougall.html

Cancer: The Cause, The Cure: Tullio Simoncini, M.D., *Cancer Is a Fungus* (Rome, Italy: Edizioni Lampis, 2007), www.cancerisafungus.com.

Otto Warburg, "The Prime Cause and Prevention of Cancer," (Lecture delivered to Nobel Laureates at Lindau, by Lake Constance, Germany, on June 30, 1966), trans and ed by Dean Burk, National Cancer Institute, p 6. Otto Warburg was the director of the Max Planck Institute for Cell Physiology, Berlin, Germany. He was the recipient of two Nobel Prizes and many other awards and honors for his work in the chemistry and physics of life. Retrieved from www.ozonetherapy.co.uk

Stephen Levine, Ph.D., and Parris M Kidd, Ph.D., "Beyond Antioxidant Adaptation: A Free Radical-Hypoxia-Clonal Thesis of Cancer Causation," *Journal of Orthomolecular Psychiatry* 14, no 3 (1985): 189–213.

Hiromi Shinya, M.D., *The Microbe Factor* (San Francisco: Council Oak Books, LLC, 2010), p 52.

Dr. Gunther Enderlein, *Blood Examination in Darkfield*, monographs summarized and trans by Dr med Maria-M Bleker (Germany: Semmelweis Verlag, 1993), p 11.

"Oxygen Therapies: Interview with Ed McCabe," by Stuart Ledbetter, *Nexus Magazine,* Aug–Sept, 1992. Adapted from an interview of Ed McCabe on NBC affiliate WPTZ Television, Plattsburgh, NY, http://www.whale.to/v/mccabe1.html

Acid Rain: Paul Withers, "New Culprit Identified in Chronic Acid Rain Problem," *CBC News* (Nova Scotia), Nov 23, 2012, http://www.cbc.ca/news/canada/nova-scotia/ story/2012/11/22/ns- acid-rain.html

Marissa Weiss, "Is Acid Rain a Thing of the Past?" June 28, 2012, http://news. sciencemag.org/sciencenow/2012/06/is-acid- rain-a-thing-of-the-past.html

Tristan Jones, "Energy, Agriculture, and the Environment: Dead Zones and the Oil Spill in the Gulf of Mexico," June 22, 2010, http://blogs.ei.columbia.edu/2010/06/22/energy-

Internal Acid Rain Theory: Garth L Nicolson, Ph.D., "Chronic Bacterial and Viral Infections in Neurodegenerative and Neurobehavioral Diseases," *Medscape,* posted June 23, 2008, http:// www.medscape.com/viewarticle/574944

Lorne Label, M.D., personal communication, 1998. Dr. Label is associate clinical professor of neurology at the David Geffen School of Medicine at UCLA, adjunct faculty at Loyola Marymount University, medical director of both the Southern California Attention Deficit Disorder Clinic and the

Brain Longevity Center, and is in private practice with California Neurological Specialists, where he practices adult and pediatric neurology and medical acupuncture.

*Pogo* is the title and central character of a comic strip created by Walt Kelly (1913– 1973).

## CHAPTER 3: HOW TO CREATE AN ALKALINE BODY

What are electrolytes: https://medlineplus.gov/fluidandelectrolytebalance.html

The four main electrolytes: https://www.ncbi.nlm.nih.gov/books/NBK541123/

Plant foods highest in electrolytes: https://www.medicalnewstoday.com/articles/electrolytes-food

## CHAPTER 4: NATURE'S FOOD CHAIN

Nature's Food Chain: https://neprimateconservancy.org/food-chain/#:~:text=THE%20FOOD%20CHAIN&text=In%20ecology%2C%20the%20food%20chain,larger%20ones%2C%20and%20so%20on.

Microbial World Within Us: https://www.harvardmagazine.com/node/76523#:~:text=The%20most%20versatile%20chemists%20in,than%20in%20our%20own%20cells.

Dr. Margaret McFall: https://mmi.wisc.edu/staff/mcfall-ngai-margaret/

Microbiome and Julie Segree, Ph.D. http://www.genome.gov/ Staff/Segre/

Dr. Will Bylsiewicz: https://zoe.com/willb?utm_source=google_pmax&utm_medium=&utm_campaign=20518243836&utm_adgroup=&utm_term=&utm_content=&gbraid=0AAAAABejleW2MgbsoQgGOZE56hHXx8uem&gclid=Cj0KCQjwtsy1BhD7ARIsAHOi4xaPSISyXI3OpE-3FJaaKupmRp6kDObodcdRfgFu4Y00KgqIS2jC0e0aAlzbEALw_wcB

DiBaise JK, Zhang H, Crowell MD, Krajmalnik-Brown R, Decker GA, Rittmann BE. Gut microbiota and its possible relationship with obesity. *Mayo Clin Proc*. 2008 Apr;83(4):460-9.

## CHAPTER 5: EAT RIGHT FOR YOUR ANATOMICAL TYPE

Homo sapiens: https://www.sciencedaily.com/releases/2012/06/120627132047.htm

Humans Are Frugivores By Nature's Design: https://frugivorebiology.com/human-frugivore-adaptations/#:~:text=Humans%20undoubtedly%20come%20from%20a,(fruit%2Deaters)%20today!

Victoria Boutenko, *Green for Life* (Ashland, OR: Raw Family Pub, 2005), p. 11.

Dr. Katherine Milton, "Diet and Primate Evolution," *Scientific American*, Aug 1993: 86–93, http://nature.berkeley.edu/miltonlab/pdfs/diet_primate_evolution.pdf

Dr. Kathrine Milton quote: (Nutrition Vol.15, No.6, 1999) Dr. Kathrine Milton: http://beforewords.net/

Carolus Linnaeus: https://fruitfest.co.uk/linnaeus/

Frances Moore Lappé, *Diet for a Small Planet* (1971; New York: Ballantine, 1991), p. 12.

Cardiologist William C. Roberts, M.D., https://prime.peta.org/news/humans-evolved-herbivores/#:~:text=As%20Dr.,beings%20are%20not%20natural%20carnivores.

Robert Morse, ND, *The Detox Miracle Sourcebook* (Prescott, AZ: Hohm Press, 2004), pp 8–11. Dr. Morse operates a natural health clinic in Florida, specializing in brain and nerve regeneration. See his website at http://www.drmorsesherbalhealthclub.com/

Dr. Herbert Shelton, N.D., author of *Superior Nutrition* quote: http://www.agedefyingbody.com/ReverseAging.html

Evidence: Were Humans Meant to Eat Meat?" *E/The Environmental Magazine* 13, no 1 ( Jan/ Febr 2002), www.emagazine.com

Hilton Hotema, *Man's Higher Consciousness* (Kessinger Publishing, 1962).

But Where Do I Get My Protein: Deborah E Sellmeyer, Katie L Stone, Anthony Sebastian, Steven R Cummings, and the Study of Osteoporotic Fractures Research Group, UNC-SF, "A High Ratio of Dietary Animal to Vegetable Protein Increases the Rate of Bone Loss and the Risk of Fracture in Postmenopausal Women," *American Journal of Clinical Nutrition* 73, no 1 ( Jan 2001): 118–22.

## CHAPTER 6: DIETARY DEVOLUTION

David L. Duffy, M.D. quote: http://en.wikipedia.org/wiki/ Arnold_Ehret

### DIETARY DEVOLUTION #1
### From Frugivore to Herbivore to Omnivore

Alan Walker: https://www.nytimes.com/1979/05/15/archives/teeth-show-fruit-was-the-staple-no-exceptions-found.html

Homo sapiens: https://www.palomar.edu/anthro/homo2/mod_homo_4.htm#:~:text=So%20far%2C%20the%20earliest%20finds,%2D40%2C000%20years%20ago.

Pre-agricultural Homo Sapiens and their Hominid Ancestors," *American Journal of Clinical Nutrition* 76, no 6 (Dec 2002): 1308–16.

Onomacritus of Athens: https://en.wikipedia.org/wiki/Onomacritus

Philochorus: https://www.attalus.org/translate/philochorus.html

Mike Anderson, *Eating*, 3rd ed (RaveDiet.com, 88 min, 2008).

## DIETARY DEVOLUTION #2
### From Omnivore to Carnivore to Chemivore

Paula Baillie-Hamilton, M.D., *The Body Restoration Plan* (New York: Penguin, 2002).

Paula Baillie-Hamilton, M.D., Ph.D., *The Body Restoration Plan: Eliminate Chemical Calories and Repair Your Body's Natural Slimming System* (New York: Penguin, 2002). This is a little-known but truly valuable resource.

Cold Cuts: Amanda J Cross, Michael F Leitzmann, Mitchell H Gail, Albert R Hollenbeck, Arthur Schatzkin, Rashmi Sinha, "A Prospective Study of Red and Processed Meat Intake in Relation to Cancer Risk," *PLoS Med* 4, no 12 (2007): e325. doi: 10.1371/ journal.pmed.0040325

CS Bruning-Fann, JB Kaneene, "The Effects of Nitrate, Nitrite, and N-nitroso Compounds on Human Health: A Review," *Vet Human Toxicology* 35 (1993): 521–38.

Nelson Mandela: https://www.britannica.com/list/nelson-mandela-quotes

Alicia Chang, "Radioactive Bluefin Tuna: Japan Nuclear Plant Contaminated Fish Found off California Coast," *Huffington Post*, May 28, 2012.

Michael Collins, "Japanese Seaweed Radiation Doubles," April 20, 2012, EnviroReporter.com.

Environmental Working Group, "Brain Food: Government Seafood Consumption Advice Could Expose 1 in 4 Newborns to Elevated Mercury Levels," April 13, 2001, http:// www.ewg.org/book/export/html/8143

HL Queen, *Chronic Mercury Toxicity: New Hope Against an Endemic Disease*

Ronald A Hites, Jeffery A Foran, David O Carpenter, M Coreen Hamilton, Barbara A Knuth, Steven J Schwager, "Global Assessment of Organic Contaminants in Farmed Salmon," *Science* 303, no 5655 (2004): 226–29, doi: 10.1126/ science.1091447

Kristen Schmitt, "Wild No More: Farm-Raised Fish labeled as 'Wild Caught'," *UrbanTimes*, April 23, 2012, http:// www.theurbn.com/2012/04/wild-no-more- farm-raised-fish- labeled-as-wild-caught/

Drugged Cows and Milk: Keith B Woodford, *Devil in the Milk: Illness, Health and Politics of A1 and A2 Milk*

(White River Junction, VT: Chelsea Green Pub, 2009). William Campbell Douglass II, M.D., *The Raw Truth about*

*Milk,* rev and expanded ed (Douglass Family Pub: 2007).

See the many articles on the dangers of milk at www.notmilk.com

Linda Joyce Forristal, CTA, MTA, "Ultra-Pasteurized Milk," May 23, 2004, www. motherlindas.com

Don Huber: https://globalearthrepairfoundation.org/don-huber-glyphosate-dangers-and-soil-remediation/

Don Huber, Transcript of interview by Dr. Joseph Mercola, Jan 2012, http:// mercola.fileburst.com/PDF/ ExpertInterviewTranscripts/ InterviewDonHuberPart2.pdf

Dave Asprey, "The Molding of the World Part 1: How We Made Mycotoxins into the Health Disaster They Are Today," March 22, 2012, http://www.bulletproofexec. com/mycotoxins- in-america/

Richard Pressinger, MEd, and Wayne Sinclair, M.D., "Researching Effects of Chemicals and Pesticides upon Health," http://www.chem-tox.com/

Mycotoxins: Charles M Benbrook, Chief Scientist, The Organic Center, "Breaking the Mold: Impacts of Organic and Conventional Farming Systems on Mycotoxins in Food and Livestock Feed," Sept2006, www.organic-center.org/reportfiles/ MycotoxinReport. pdf

Irradiated Foods: Organic Consumers Association, "What's Wrong with Food Irradiation," Feb 2001, http://www.organicconsumers.org/Irrad/irradfact.cfm

Organic Consumers Association, "Status Update on Food Irradiation," July 5, 2002, http://www.organicconsumers.org/ Irrad/status.cfm

Monsanto GMO: Joe Cummins, "Bt Toxins in Genetically Modified Crops: Regulation by Deceit," Institute of Science in Society, March 23, 2004, http://www.i-sis.org.uk/BTTIGMC. php

Dag Falck, "Does the Current Organic Practice Standard Adequately Address GMO Contamination?" *The Organic and Non-GMO Report,* Jan 2008, http:// www.non-gmoreport.com/ articles/jan08/organic_practice_ standard_and_gmo_ contamination.ph

Relaena, "Is Organic Always GMO Free?" *GMO Awareness,* May 5, 2011, http:// gmo-awareness.com/2011/05/05/is- organic-always-gmo-free/

"What Are the Dangers?" Mothers for Natural Law, http:// www.safe-food.org/- issue/dangers.html

"Arpad Pusztain and the Risks of Genetic Engineering," *The Organic and Non-GMO Report,* ed Ken Roseboro, 2009.

Barry Flamm, Chair of the National Organic Standards Board, "Open Letter from National Organic Standards Board to USDA on GMO Contamination of Organic Crops," March 28, 2012, http://www.organicconsumers.org/articles/article_25217. cfm

How to read the stickers on your produce to avoid GMOs: Dr. Frank Lipman,

http://www.drfranklipman.com/what-do-those-codes-on- stickers-of-fruits-and- some-veggies-mean/

Joël Spiroux de Vendômois, Francois Roullier, Dominique Cellier, Gilles-Eric Séralini, "A Comparison of the Effects of Three GM Corn Varieties on Mammalian Health," *Int J Biological Sciences* 5, no 7 (2009): 706–26, doi: 10.7150/ ijbs.5.706

Rady Ananda, "Three Approved GMOs Linked to Organ Damage," Jan 3, 2012, http://prn.fm/2012/01/03/foodfreedom- com-three-approved-gmos-linked-to- organ-damage/ #axzz1wZmHPTF4

Michael Pollan, interview by Amy Goodman, *Democracy Now,* Oct 24, 2012. For a transcript see http:// www.democracynow.org/2012/10/24/ michael_pollan_ californias_prop_37_fight

## DIETARY DEVOLUTION #3
### From Chemivore to Junkivore to Drugivore

Economic Research Service, Table 13: US Per Capita Food Expenditures, http:// www.ers.usda.gov/data-products/food- expenditures.aspx

David U Himmelstein, M.D., Deborah Thorne, Ph.D, Elizabeth Warren, JD, Steffie Woolhandler, N.D., MPH, "Medical Bankruptcy in the United States, 2007: Results of a National Study," *American Journal of Medicine* 20, no 10 (2009), doi: 10.1016/j. amjmed.2009.04.012

Empty Calories: Mark Hyman, M.D., "How Malnutrition Causes Obesity," *Huffington Post,* March 8, 2012, http:// www.huffingtonpost.com/dr-mark-hyman/malnutrition- obesity_b_1324760.html and "Skinny Fat People: Why Being Skinny Doesn't Protect Us Against Diabetes and Death," May 22, 2012, http://drhyman.com/blog/2012/05/22/skinny-fat- people-why-being-skinny-doesnt-protect-us-againstdiabetes- and-death/

Fake Foods: K He, L Zhao, ML Daviglus, AR Dyer, L Van Horn, D Garside, L Zhu, D Guo, Y Wu, B Zhou, J Stamler; INTERMAP Cooperative Research Group, "Association of Monosodium Glutamate Intake with Overweight in Chinese Adults: the INTERMAP Study," *Obesity (Silver Spring)* 16, no 8 (2008): 1875–80.

Fake Sugar: Janet Starr Hull, Creator of the Aspartame Detox Program, "Dangers of Aspartame Poisoning," 2002, www.sweetpoison.com/aspartame-information.html

Janet Starr Hull, Creator of the Aspartame Detox Program, "Dangers of Aspartame Poisoning," 2002, www.sweetpoison.com/aspartame-information.html

Lendon H Smith, M.D., "ADHD and ADD: The Hyperactive Child," http://www.phosadd.com/support%20evidence/lsmithhtm

Theresa Dale, ND, "Aspartame: More Unsavory Side Effects," *Spartan of Truth: Archive for Lendon Smith, M.D.,* Dec 4, 2011, http://spartanoftruth.wordpress.com/tag/lendon-smith-m-d/

Sandra Cabot, M.D., "Aspartame Makes You Fatter!" Position Statement, July 22, 2006, http://www.liverdoctor.com

Dangers of Fake Meat: https://www.hsph.harvard.edu/news/hsph-in-the-news/plant-based-meat-health/#:~:text="Some%20of%20those%20products%2C%20even,t%20necessarily%20mean%20it's%20healthier."

Dangers of Fake Fat: Myra Karstadt and Stephen Schmidt, "Olestra: Procter's Big Gamble," *CSPI Nutrition Action Health Letter,* March 1996, http://www.cspinet.org/olestra/pbg.html

Susan E Swithers, Sean B Ogden, Terry L Davidson, "Fat Substitutes Promote Weight Gain in Rats consuming high-fat diets," *Behavioral Neuroscience* 125, no 4 (Aug 2011): 512–18, doi: 10.1037/a0024404

Melinda Wenner, "Humans Carry More Bacterial Cells than Human Ones," *Scientific American,* Nov 30, 2007, http:// www.scientificamerican.com/article. cfm?id=strange-but-true- humans-carry-more-bacterial-cells-than-human-ones

George J Armelagos, Kathleen C Barnes, and James Lin, "Disease in Human Evolution: The Re-Emergence of Infections Disease in the Third Epidemiological Transition," *National Museum of Natural History Bulletin for Teachers* 18, no 3 (Fall 1996).

Colorado Springs, CO: Queen and Company Health Communications, 1988). Bernard Jensen, D.C., N.D., Ph.D., *Iridology: Science and Practice in the Healing Arts, Vol II* (Escondido, CA: Bernard Jensen, 1982), p 436–37.

Disease in Human Evolution: https://moodle2.units.it/pluginfile.php/315068/mod_resource/content/0/Disease%20in%20Human%20Evolution-%20The%20Re-Emergence%20of%20Infectious%20Disease%20in%20the%20Third%20Epidemiological%20Transition.pdf

A Tale of Two Cities: https://dickens.ucsc.edu/programs/dickens-to-go/best-of-times.html

## PART TWO – THE RETURN

## CHAPTER 7: ENLIGHTEN YOURSELF WITH NATURE'S FOUR FUEL GROUPS

### Earth: Eat to Enlighten Yourself

Photosynthesis: https://education.nationalgeographic.org/resource/photosynthesis/

Phytochemicals/nutrients: https://www.uclahealth.org/news/article/what-are-phytochemicals-and-why-should-you-eat-more-them

Debbie Krivitsky on phytochemicals: https://www.health.harvard.edu/staying-healthy/fill-up-on-phytochemicals

American Institute for Cancer Research: https://www.aicr.org/resources/blog/healthtalk-whats-the-difference-between-an-antioxidant-and-a-phytochemical/

Andrea Murray: https://www.mdanderson.org/publications/focused-on-health/5-benefits-of-a-plant-based-diet.h20-1592991.html

Stanford Medicine studies: https://web.stanford.edu/group/nutrition/cgi-bin/pbdi/wordpress/

Foods highest in phytochemicals: https://stanfordhealthcare.org/medical-clinics/cancer-nutrition-services/reducing-cancer-risk/phytochemicals.html

Electric Universe: https://rationalwiki.org/wiki/Electric_Universe

Electric Universe book by Wallace Thornhill: https://www.stickmanonstone.com/shop/p/electricuniverse

Michael Hickner: https://www.livescience.com/62570-potato-battery-conduct-electricity.html#

Dr. Robert Morse: https://www.earthsongfarm.com/WellBeingFruits.htm

UCLA mitochondria: https://medschool.ucla.edu/news-article/mitochondria-function-form-and-food#:~:text=(That%20they%20work%20much%20like,different%20parts%20of%20a%20cell.

## Air: Breathe to Enlighten Yourself

The Breath Affect: https://www.thebreatheffect.com/the-power-of-your-breath/

The Healing Effects of Deep Breathing: https://www.wsj.com/articles/the-healing-power-of-proper-breathing-11590098696

The Power of Deep Breathing: https://positivepsychology.com/deep-breathing-techniques-exercises/

## Fire: Sunbathe to Enlighten Yourself

Michael Holick, M.D: https://drmichaelholick.org/wp-content/uploads/2021/11/Sunlight-and-Vitamin-D.pdf

https://www.ncbi.nlm.nih.gov/pmc/articles/PMC3738435/

https://pubmed.ncbi.nlm.nih.gov/20398766/

National Library of Medicine: https://www.ncbi.nlm.nih.gov/pmc/articles/PMC2290997/

https://www.ncbi.nlm.nih.gov/pmc/articles/PMC7400257/

Sunlight Exposure and Microbiome: https://www.medicalnewstoday.com/articles/326782

Nathan, Bryan, PHD, https://pubmed.ncbi.nlm.nih.gov/35636654/

https://d.newswise.com/articles/new-study-by-nathan-bryan-phd-explains-why-the-early-formation-of-nitric-oxide-in-the-mouth-by-oral-bacteria-is-essential-to-health-including-the-management-of-blood-pressure

Prof. Bruce Vallance: https://pubmed.ncbi.nlm.nih.gov/31708890/

Researcher Elsa Bosman: https://www.nbcnews.com/health/health-news/how-sun-exposure-can-affect-your-microbiome-n1071021

https://www.medicalnewstoday.com/articles/326782

Sungazing benefits and precautions: https://www.healthline.com/health/mind-body/sun-gazing

Phytochemicals Protect UV Damage: https://www.researchgate.net/figure/Examples-of-phytochemicals-that-protect-against-damage-by-UV-radiation_fig1_23164995#:~:text=Phenolic%20compounds%2C%20alkaloids%20and%20carotenoids,skin%20cancers%20and%20related%20illnesses.

https://www.sciencedirect.com/science/article/abs/pii/S1568163720302622#:~:text=Phytochemicals%20prevent%20extracellular%20degradation%20and,apoptosis%2C%20DNA%20damages%20and%20immunosuppression.

## Water: Drink to Enlighten Yourself

The Early Earth: https://new.nsf.gov/news/scientists-determine-early-earth-was-water-world#:~:text=The%20Earth%20of%203.2%20billion,origin%20of%20life%20on%20Earth.

Ionization Energy: https://chem.libretexts.org/Bookshelves/Physical_and_Theoretical_Chemistry_Textbook_Maps/Supplemental_Modules_(Physical_and_Theoretical_Chemistry)/Physical_Properties_of_Matter/Atomic_and_Molecular_Properties/Ionization_Energy

Hydrogen-rich Water: https://www.ncbi.nlm.nih.gov/pmc/articles/PMC6307663/

Water is H2O: https://www.scientificamerican.com/article/why-does-combining-hydrog/

Dehydration: https://my.clevelandclinic.org/health/diseases/9013-dehydration

Dr. Mu Shik John: https://naturalactionwater.ca/research/dr-mu-shik-jhon/

F. Batmanghelidj, M.D., Author of Your Body's Many Cries for Water, You're Not Sick, You're Thirsty: https://en.wikipedia.org/wiki/Fereydoon_Batmanghelidj

CDC Report: https://www.cdc.gov/healthywater/drinking/public/understanding_ccr.html

EPA: https://www.epa.gov/newsreleases/biden-harris-administration-finalizes-first-ever-national-drinking-water-standard

Benefits of Detox Baths: https://www.thestewartcenterforoptimalhealth.com/2021/02/03/benefits-of-detox-baths/

Benefits of Hot and Cold Therapy: https://www.uclahealth.org/news/article/6-cold-shower-benefits-consider

https://www.physiotattva.com/therapies/hot-and-cold-therapy#:~:text=Combining%20heat%20and%20ice%20therapy,for%20treating%20pain%20and%20discomfort.

Benefits of Colon Hydrotherapy: https://www.webmd.com/balance/natural-colon-cleansing-is-it-necessary

# ABOUT THE AUTHOR

Toni Toney earned her "master's degree" from the highest possible school of learning: NATURE! After almost dying, she discovered that the foods she had been eating had created what we call dis-ease.

The *New Earth Diet* is the food program that Toni subscribed to when medicine failed to help her. Her purpose in writing this book is that it might help you, too. After traveling the world for answers, Toni came to realize that our diseases are merely a reflection of the diseases of the planet; that the root cause of almost every disease is simply the type of food we "burn for fuel" into our body's internal environment. The recipes in this book were artistically and favorably created by her over the years when she owned an organic vegan restaurant.

As the creator of the New Earth Times message, she is inviting you to join her in a movement whose time has come—the quest to prepare our physical bodies for the shift of the ages by infusing it with lots of LIGHT through the foods we eat!

Welcome to one of the most life-changing, revolutionary cookbooks of our time! It offers us a way of eating that produces LIGHT within our physical bodies through the power of phytochemical/nutrients created by the power of the sun—plant foods that ENLIGHTEN US!

*Bon Apetite!*

With love,
Toni Toney

tonitoney.com

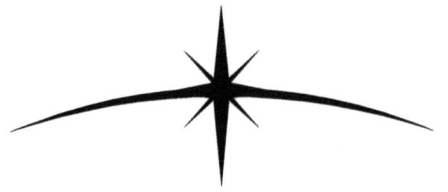

www.ingramcontent.com/pod-product-compliance
Lightning Source LLC
LaVergne TN
LVHW061034070526
838201LV00073B/5035